Representations of the Body in French Renaissance Poetry

Studies in the Humanities
Literature—Politics—Society

Guy Mermier
General Editor

Vol. 47

PETER LANG
New York • Washington, D.C./Baltimore • Boston
Bern • Frankfurt am Main • Berlin • Vienna • Paris

Karen R. Sorsby

Representations of the Body in French Renaissance Poetry

PETER LANG
New York • Washington, D.C./Baltimore • Boston
Bern • Frankfurt am Main • Berlin • Vienna • Paris

Library of Congress Cataloging-in-Publication Data

Sorsby, Karen R.
Representations of the body in French Renaissance poetry / Karen R. Sorsby.
p. cm. — (Studies in the humanities; vol. 47)
Includes bibliographical references and index.
1. French poetry—16th century—History and criticism. 2. Body, Human, in literature. 3. Sex in literature. 4. Aesthetics in literature. 5. Literature and medicine—France—History—16th century. I. Title. II. Series: Studies in the humanities (New York, N.Y.); vol. 47.
PQ418.S67 841'.30936—dc21 98-36826
ISBN 0-8204-4267-4
ISSN 0742-6712

Die Deutsche Bibliothek-CIP-Einheitsaufnahme

Sorsby, Karen R.:
Representations of the body in French renaissance poetry / Karen R. Sorsby.
–New York; Washington, D.C./Baltimore; Boston; Bern;
Frankfurt am Main; Berlin; Vienna; Paris: Lang.
(Studies in the humanities; Vol. 47)
ISBN 0-8204-4267-4

Front cover photo used with the permission
of Blocker History of Medicine Collections, Moody Medical Library,
The University of Texas Medical Branch at Galveston.

The paper in this book meets the guidelines for permanence and durability
of the Committee on Production Guidelines for Book Longevity
of the Council of Library Resources.

Printed in the United States of America

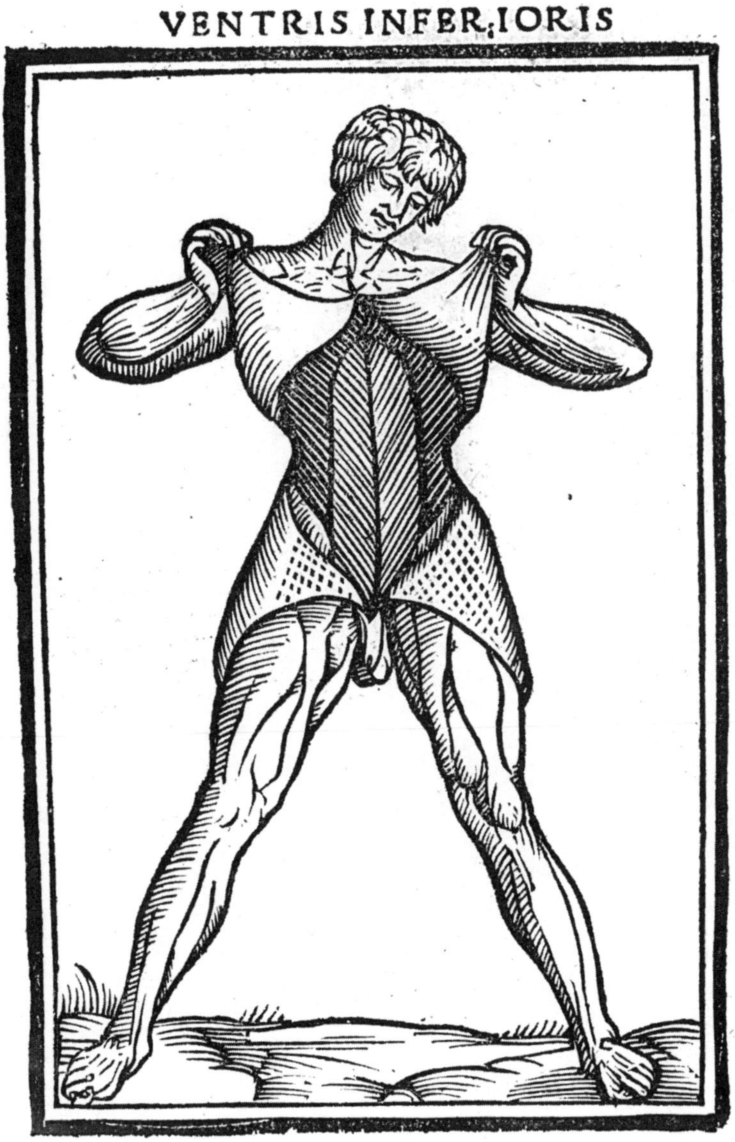

A dissection of thoracic muscles, *ventris inferioris*, from Jacopo Berengario, *Anatomia Carpi. Isagoge breves, perlucide ac uberime, in anatomiam humani corporis*, Venetiis, Bernardinum De Vitalibus, 1535. (Photo Courtesy of the National Library of Medicine, Bethesda.)

Table of Contents

Illustrations

Introduction

The French Renaissance was a period of rapid and radical change that engendered reexaminations and redefinitions in all fields of learning. The ultimate object of enquiry was veritable knowledge, particularly about man's physical body, his nature, his soul, his world and his universe.[1]

Renaissance philosophers, theologians, physicians, poets and others nurtured a shared goal of understanding man. Humanistic values, which emphasized classical purity of language and sources, transformed anatomy and poetry. Inspired by classical forms and models, poets developed a new poetry. Theologians and philosophers, contemplating "l'excellence des oeuvres de Dieu,"[3] considered man's body to be the reflection of the Christian tradition, a conveyor of religious intentions and actions. Conversely, the woman's body was often treated as the "weaker vessel" in biblical texts (Gen. 2:21, I Pet. 3:7), and thus often represented as an imperfect or incomplete version of the male.[3]

Renaissance anatomists cited inaccuracies in Galen's anatomy to demonstrate that his work was essentially worthless because of his failure to perform human dissections. The conclusion was skillfully chronicled by Charles Estienne in a treatise in which he emphasized that doctors should gain knowledge of the human body through dissection.

> . . . luy est requis & necessaire . . . la congnoissance des parties tant interieures qu'exterieures du corps humain: et ce/par frequentes dissections . . . non pas de corps de singes. . . . Ne vouldrions pareillement lesdictes anatomies estre faictes de corps de chiens/ou pourceaulx. . . . Mais vouldrions lesdites exertations anatomiques estre faictes sur les corps d'hommes ou de femmes.[4]

The combined inquiries of physicians, philosophers, theologians, poets and artists led to a more accurate representation of the human body. Physicians judiciously began to practice public anatomies during the second half of the sixteenth century, usually on males.[5] Philosophers and theologians reflected on the essence of man and his relationship to the universe, as did poets. Artists refined the use of perspective developed a century earlier in Italy. There was much speculation about the physical composition of the human body, whose external unity and internal diversity formed natural subjects for poetic expression.

Poets examined in this study were profoundly, even obsessively, concerned with representing body's material composition. Each explores the encounter between the power of poetic language and the objects that he is trying to represent. Each is preoccupied with disclosing basic aspects of the body in poetic language rather than merely describing it in prose.

Sixteenth-century French poets considered the acquisition of self-knowledge to be necessary to the understanding of man, *le petit monde*. They relied on anatomy in their poetry to provide a sense of body and soul that they believed to be necessary to acquire that knowledge. This study explores Renaissance poets' representations of the male and female body as a material construct by defining the body's anatomy as the poets did, by interpreting its meaning within the framework of Renaissance poetry and historical change, and by linking its representations to the growth of the concept of self.

The image of the body constantly evolved in both poetry and medicine during the sixteenth century. Poetic theory, poetry, and anatomical inquiry underwent similar restructuring, reflecting both a rejection of medieval forms and an increasing interest in structure and composition. Renaissance poetry, particularly scientific poetry, became encyclopedic in nature. It projected a desire to compile and define terms relating to the infinite variety of marvelous phenomena in the universe. The importance French poetic theorists gave to the human body in their treatises is apparent in their repeated linkage of it to two fundamental and interrelated literary preoccupations: the rehabilitation and enrichment of the French language, and the quest for gaining self-knowledge by contemplating body. Their allusions to the body emanated from a desire to draw on the considerable resources of the language to write better poetry while also enriching the poetic vocabulary with new words and forms of expression. To accomplish these goals, Pierre de Ronsard, in his *Abbregé de l'Art poëtique françois* (1565), advised poets to familiarize themselves with the handiwork of artisans to further embellish their own work. He used the lexicon of the body to capture poetic inventions as flesh and blood constructs, and cited explicit examples of the human body to renew poetic discourse.

> car tout ainsi qu'on ne peut pas dire un corps humain beau, plaisant & accomply, s'il n'est composé de sang, venes arteres & tendrons, & surtout d'une nayve couleur. Ainsi la Poesie ne peut estre si plaisante, vive ne parfaite sans belles inventions, descriptions, comparaisons, qui font les ners & la vie du

livre . . . .[6]

Ronsard's suggestion that the body is a source of vitality in poetry illustrates his desire to explore the potentialities of the sensible and tangible universe. With this objective in mind, the present work seeks to gain insight into the practices of selected Renaissance poets and to delineate the diversity of viewpoints in representing the image of the human body in their work. They described the body using new models borrowed from other genres, particularly art, medicine and religion.

Chapter I
Poets of the Creation

Creation, the supreme moment in Judeo-Christian origins, is a common subject in French Renaissance poetry. Poets who drew inspiration from Genesis adhered to the biblical account of Creation to varying degrees; some of them interpreted Genesis closely, others more broadly, yet each was unique in his use of vocabulary and forms of expression, and thus each visualized the body *sui generis*. This chapter is devoted to works by several poets who drew their inspiration from Genesis and the six days of Creation and one short anatomical poem based on the aftermath of the Fall. I examine how these poets departed from the biblical account by dissecting man's body on a rational and scientific plane, while continuing to use Creation as a narrative grounding to provide cosmological, medical and anatomical representations of God's wondrous creation. Various factors led to the popular movement towards poetically dissecting man's body, although poetic license alone provides some explanation for it.

I focus mainly on the Renaissance interest in anatomical science and cosmology and the encyclopedism which contributed greatly to the perspective of the poetry of the body. Poets found inspiration to poeticize the body within these disciplines, which were often linked to music, painting and artistic creation generally.

Several related topics are of considerable interest, but they fall outside the scope of this study. These include the treatment of Creation historically in Renaissance poetic texts, the origin of mankind described therein, and how these texts parallel Genesis in presenting a biblical view of the body of man.

The Microcosm

> Man is called by the ancients a world in miniature and certainly this name is well applied, for just as man is composed of earth, water, air and fire, so is the body of the earth. If man has in him bones which are the support and armor of the flesh, the world has rocks which are the support the earth; if man has in himself the sea of blood, in which the lungs rise and fall in breathing, so the body of the earth has its oceanic sea which also rises and falls every six hours for the world to breathe.
>
> Leonardo da Vinci[7]

> Man is heaven and earth, and lower spheres, and the four elements, and whatever is within them, wherefore he is properly called by the name of microcosmos for he is the whole world. . . . Know then that there is also within man a starry firmament with a mighty course of planets and stars that have exaltations, conjunctions and oppositions.
>
> Paracelsus[8]

The body was commonly referred to during the Middle Ages and the Renaissance as *le petit monde* (the little world, or microcosm), which corresponded in structure to the universe (the macrocosm). The premise that man's body is composed of all the elements in the universe and obeys the same laws is one of the simplest forms of the microcosmic concept, and helps to define the essence of man and his relationship to the universe.[9] Man thus serves as a link between the celestial sphere and the sublunary world.[10] Renaissance literature is replete with descriptive symbols that liken parts of the body to objects in the universe, thereby providing ways for comprehending the infinite by studying the miniature. Much of the inspiration for depicting man as microcosm was derived from ancient Greek doctrines and was transmitted through Medieval sources to the Renaissance. However, as A.-M. Schmidt observes, this conventional Medieval view of man as a microcosm was largely unmodified by Renaissance humanists:

> Les penseurs humanistes passent à l'envie leur temps à répéter les thèses d'Honoré d'Autun, affirment, pour conclure, comme lui ou Alain de Lille, que le petit monde renferme toutes les formes d'être qui parent le grand monde.[11]

During the later Renaissance some observers, notably Montaigne, criticized the use of the microcosm-macrocosm analogy in referring to man, his world, and the universe. He ridiculed philosophers for presumptuously attempting to correlate the two. Montaigne believed that "le corps a une grand' part à nostre estre," and also that ". . . sa structure et composition sont de bien juste consideration."[12] He observed that the perception of man as a microcosm, which was widely used to understand the body, permeated contemporary thought and writing. But he affirmed that the concept provided neither an accurate account nor useful description of man because it was inapplicable to any creature so vain, diverse, and inconstant.[13] Montaigne insisted that it was impossible to comprehend the true essence of the physical nature of man's body by using a microcosmic theory despite the efforts of so many philosophers, physicians, theologians and poets. He believed that the most important knowledge man could gain was self-knowledge, although he doubted that self-knowledge and knowledge of man were synonymous.[14] Nevertheless, the microcosmic influence remained strong in the mainstream of philosophical and scientific thought and continued to be a common theme in poetry.

Poets held a preeminent place in Montaigne's thoughts because they said "everything they want with more emphasis and grace" (II:37). He considered himself to be an expert on the subject, being, he boasted, "familiar enough with poetry to be a judge" (I:31). Concerning philosophy, which he called sophisticated poetry, and the philosophical contemplation of the composition of the human body, he mused in the *Apologie de Raimond Sebond* on the comparative natures of the heavenly bodies and the body of man.[15]

> Il n'y a pas plus de retrogradation, trepidation, accession, reculement, ravissement, aux astres et corps celestes, qu'ils ont forgé en ce pauvre petit corps humain. Vrayment ils ont eu par là raison de l'appeler le petit monde, tant ils ont employé de pièces et de visages à le maçonner et bastir . . . à combien d'ordres et estages ont-ils départy ce pauvre homme, outre les naturels et perceptibles? . . . Ils en font une chose publique imaginaire. C'est un sujet qu'ils tiennent et qu'ils manient: on leur laisse toute puissance de le descoudre, renger, rassembler et estoffer, chacun à sa fantasie; et si ne le possedent pas encore.[16]

The poets that I examine in the following pages of this study provide impressive examples of the kind of tasks Montaigne alludes to as they enthusiastically examine the human body "chacun à sa fantasie." They explore the analogy of the human body with the cosmos, fusing elements with the structures of the body that are conventionally associated with the macrocosm. Much of this is traditional, as has been noted. Its origins are to be found in Classical and Medieval literature; Renaissance poets introduced little that was innovative.[17] However, the enrichment of the theme through the Creation myth, which endowed it with theological dignity, and the representation of Adam and Eve as microcosmic models, are of sixteenth century origin.

Specifically, I examine references to the microcosm in representations of man's body in poems by three Creation poets (Scève, Du Bartas, D'Aubigné) and two physician-poets (Béroalde De Verville and Du Chesne). I also explore their attempts to depict both men's and women's bodies in a theological discourse with "emphasis and grace." These poets drew their inspiration from microcosmic theories that assumed that the body could serve as a standard of measurement for the "corporeal" universe because it was in absolute balance and therefore perfect. They used the body and the universe as models of each other, advancing the thesis that the elements in the human body are derived from the cosmos. In their search for ultimate truth, they made fine distinctions between the macrocosm and microcosm, implying that "The thing that is on high is like the thing that is below;"[18] if one knows the universe, or man, one knows the other. However, each poet studied here framed the body as a microcosm from a different perspective. Each fashioned it into an idealistic abstraction to create a realm of transcendence and immortality in its form and to place it within the infinite cycle of the universe.

In the poems examined below, Scève discourses on the philosophical or metaphysical aspects of the microcosm while Du Bartas explores the body poetically in the manner of a Renaissance cosmographer. D'Aubigné examines the body in a quasi-medical fashion, yet he explores the mystery of the union of the flesh and spirit. His verses are interspersed with philosophical reflections on the body as the vessel of the soul. Béroalde De Verville employs alchemical vocabulary as a vital part of a poem that focuses on the mineral composition of the cosmos and microcosmos, but which also examines the woman and her social identity. Du Chesne, rather than offering the expected medical discourse, presents a post-Adamic Fall view of a body that he believed harbored evil, debilitating passions.

1. The Poet-Metaphysician, Maurice Scève: *Microcosme* (1562)

Scève's *Microcosme* was one of the first of several lengthy sixteenth century poems that describe Creation. As Saulnier suggests, it is an excellent early example of the humanist cultural movement in France.[19] And yet while the *Microcosme* inspired creation poets later in the century, it furnishes little technical, anatomical or other scientific information concerning the structure and fabric of the body.

My examination of the poem focuses primarily on the first book (of three), which deals with Creation, the nature of man's body, the creation of Eve, and the division of the sexes. I also examine Scève's curiosity about the microcosmic concept and the importance he attaches to self-knowledge.

Scève stresses the human body's propensity for movement, which he attributes to *le grand Ouvrier* (Bk. I,v. 103), the divine Creator "Qui firent ce corps vif bouger, mouvoir, courir" (Bk. I, v.131). He portrays man in astrological terms as a microcosm emphasizing a zodiacal system of relationships between cosmography and the elements of anatomy. (Each of the twelve signs of the Zodiac corresponds to and affects a different part of the body [Fig. 1.1., Zodiac Man].)[20]

Aux Signes assignant diversité puissante:
Chauds, secs humides, froids, mais par divers accors
Matrisent regardant chacun sa part du corps,

(Bk III, vv. 366–68)

Scève uses Adam in his system of cosmography to symbolize man's body, which he presents as an inverted tree. "Teste en pié racineux, . . . cest arbre renversé. . . . Tiré des cieux cy bas. . . . Dressé sur piés branchus. . . ."[21] The body possesses the same characteristics as the universe. Consequently, its nature is determined by the physical similarities between the cosmos and all the organisms that inhabit both. Woman appears metaphorically from this celestial tree, as a wondrous birth, a branch gradually emerging from the *costé fendu* of Adam's benumbed body. Her spherical head and undulating tresses are harmonious with the shape of the earth and its aqueous element.

Et le corps assoupi, peu à peu se haussant
Une teste formee, et en sfere croissant
Couverte d'or filé, mais deliément blond
Espars, et ondoyant dessus maint membre rond
Col, espaules, et bras, gorge blanche avancee
Couvrant en son secret la pudique pensee
Enflee de deux tetins de mignonne rondeur,
Nourrissiers attrayans Amour à sa grandeur,
Le ventre ample, et fecond, double hanche, et ceinture
Du Ceste virginal rebellant à Nature
Son entree celant sous un moussu verger,

(Bk I, vv. 171–81)

Although Scève's work is not uniquely linked to religious or philosophical traditions, he draws extensively from philosophical reasoning and the Bible (Genesis 1:26–7, 2:22–3) to provide the narrative ground for depicting the creation of the human body. Adam is "Ce Microcosme vif en sa pure innocence" (Bk. I, v.147), the original human microcosmic model containing all the elements of the earth. He is inscribed as the central component within the sphere of the heavens in a world made for man. Scève preserves metaphorically the biblical notion of the woman's body as being inferior because of its different members and functions.[22] He portrays her as the *pudique* division of the sexes and also as a vision of God's magnificent work. She has a "Forme elegante, et propre au Dormant tressemblable" (v. 187). But as his use of *tressemblable* suggests, she was not fully equal to man. In Scève's systematic account of

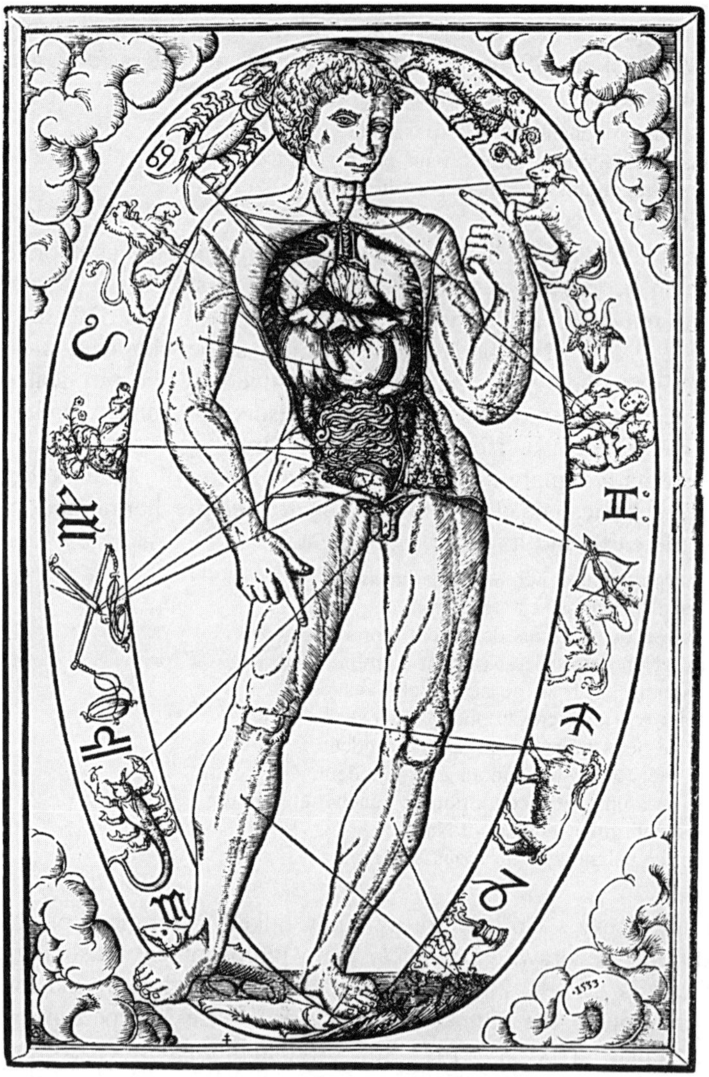

Figure 1.1 Zodiac Man, *Icy te sont represent les douze signes Zodiaque ayans domination sur les parties que tu voys particulierement marquées.* Charles Estienne, *Les figures et portraicts des parties du corps humain*, Paris, I. Kerver, ca. 1575. Plates taken from Estienne's *De dissectione partium corporis humani* (Paris, 1546). (Photo: Courtesy of the Blocker History of Medicine Collections, Moody Medical Library, The University of Texas Medical Branch at Galveston.)

Adam and Eve's creation, the procreation of the female, particularly, reveals the poet's understanding of the concepts of sexual differences and the status of woman. The features of her more voluptuous body suggest her inner character and generative capacities. Accordingly, her figure is shown as being fashioned of

> . . . maint membre rond
> Col, espaules, et bras, gorge blanche avancee
> . . .
> . . . deux tetins de mignonne rondeur,
> Nourrissiers attrayans Amour à sa grandeur,
> Le ventre ample, et fecond, double hanche, . . .
>
> (Bk I, 174–75, 77–79)

The male's body is aptly suited to physical labor, with strong, protruding, root like and flexible limbs. It is formed of

> . . . deux flancs en branches . . .
> Distinctes de rameaux et noueux, et flechibles
> Pour aptes instruments à tous labeurs possibles.
> . . . ce Modelle si beau . . .
> Fut solidé en os vestus de chair, et peau.
>
> (Bk I, 114–116, 125–26)

Except for drawing microcosmic and Genesis parallels, Scève makes no in-depth examination of the body's anatomical structure or composition. There is little evidence of the contemporary anatomical inquiry such as that found in the poems of Du Bartas or D'Aubigné. The questions of the extent of Scève's interest in acquiring knowledge of the body and portraying its visual image poetically are linked closely to religious discourse and to artistic aspiration, as is his desire for self-knowledge. Scève acknowledges that the body, as an object of representation, must be interpreted primarily within the context of divine artistic inspiration. He seeks this inspiration to enable him to describe and praise God's masterpiece.

> De ton divin Esprit enflamme mon courage
> Pour descrire ton Homme, et louër ton ouvrage,
> Ouvrage vrayement Chef d'oeuvre de ta main:
> A ton image fait et divin, et humain.
>
> (Bk I, 3–6)

Several Creation poets examined in this study not only represented the body as a microcosm, and interpreted it within the context of divine artistic inspiration, but they also drew comparisons between the "sister arts" of poetry and art, each of which venerates the body. They understood the affinity between the two arts and the powerful creative stimuli in each, in which poets and artists alike sought to instruct and to please their readers (in words) or viewers (on the canvas) about that which is observable about the body. In his preface to the *Microcosme*, Scève succinctly describes his intention to please the reader.

Ainsi errant dessous ce cours Solaire
Tardif je tasche inutile à te plaire
Ne mendiant de toi autre faveur.

Du Bartas also recognized the importance of the arts and their fundamental significance to a poem's structure and, ultimately, to the reader. He provides a clear indication of his poetic and artistic objectives in depicting the body. It is to his examination of the human body that we now turn.

2. The Poet-Cosmographer, Guillaume De Saluste Sieur Du Bartas: *Première semaine*, *Le sixième jour de la sepmaine* (1578)

Du Bartas presents a common—but essential—Renaissance view of man as *le petit monde* in the following verses from *Le sixième jour*, in which he uses the example of the body as *l'humain bastiment*, *un abregé du monde*, and *Un tableau racourci* of that world.

IL N'Y A (comme dit l'un des Bessons de Dele)
Sous la voute du Ciel, conoissance plus belle
Que celle de soy-mesme: on ne trouve argument
Plus fecond en discours que l'humain bastiment.
En nous se void le feu, l'air, et la terre et l'onde:
Et bref l'homme n'est rien qu'un abregé du monde,
Un tableau racourci, que sur l'autre Univers
Je veux ore tirer du pinceau de mes vers

(*Le sixième jour*, vv. 401–8)[23]

Just as Scève did, Du Bartas acknowledged the importance of self-knowledge and artistic inspiration in exploring and understanding this microcosmic body. He also affirmed that man's body, being composed of the four elements (air, water, fire and earth), mirrored the universe, or macrocosm. Du Bartas asserted that the soul, in contrast to the body, possessed none of these elements, but consisted rather of a *cinquiseme essence* (v.711), whose nature "Fuye nos foibles yeux: . . ." (v.756). It is "Non-fini, non-mortel, non-meslé, non-palpable" (v.760), and possesses the agile capacity to relocate itself throughout the microcosm, "Soit tout en tout le corps, et tout en chasque part, Soit qu'il regne au cerveau, soit au coeur il habite" (vv.760–61).[24]

But unlike Scève, who analyzed man in terms of his zodiacal correspondence with the macrocosm and by botanical analogies, Du Bartas conceived of the human body as a geographical region through which he could journey, thereby implying that he played an important role as the body's cosmographer. He could thus objectively contemplate the body and, with God's grace, its affiliation both to the terrestrial world and to the cosmos. He acknowledged that being a poet-cosmographer required skill, and that his task was a formidable one because the body and the universe were ordered wholes of immense complexity. Thus mapping the features of the body was as difficult as mapping the terrestrial and celestial worlds. Du Bartas, in common with other poets, was unable to see the whole design simultaneously and represented only part of it at a time. But he had faith that a comprehensive design did exist and attempted to control the total unity of this "fleshy house" while dividing it into its constituent parts.

Du Bartas maintained exacting standards in describing the body's anatomical, cosmographical and geographical features, yet he intentionally provided the reader with only a selective and superficial view of these features (vv. 699–700). He thereby avoided having to deal with the entire cosmographical and anatomical conception of the body, while preserving the integrity and focus of his role as poet.

Du Bartas reveals the discoveries made on this *grand voyage* through the body that he began as a way to acquire self-knowledge ("conoissance . . . de soy-mesme"). In addition, the comparisons that he draws between painting and poetry provide a clearer view of the elements of the human body that must be painted or "drawn out" (*tirer du pinceau*) by the poet's artistic craft. Yet while he is so concerned with representing in verse the image of this little world, he depicts the body's anatomy unrealistically, invariably exaggerating its structure in idealized cosmographical overtones.

Du Bartas' scrutiny of the body is largely unaccompanied by experimental verification, although he does suggest in several important verses that it be opened by a surgeon's scalpel (an operation described below under the title of poet-prosector). Apart from this expressed desire for anatomical confirmation, he bases his inquiry on classical studies of anatomy. He admits that his examination of the body is only mediocre in comparison to the perspicacious work of learned men such as Galen, Aesculapius, and Herophilus. Nevertheless, while acknowledging their stature, he concluded that God should be the ultimate authority, and so rejected them to further his own poetic endeavor. And so, primarily to demonstrate God's power's, he explored the body poetically *par . . . eschantillon* (in representative samples).

> Mais non, je ne veux pas faire une ample reveue
> Des membres que l'ouvrier desrobe à nostre veue.
> Car ce brave projet requiert la docte main
> Des deux fils d'AEsculape, et le labouré style
> Du disert Galien, ou du haut Herophile.

Par cest eschantillon il me suffit d'avoir
Tellement quellement monstré le sainct pouvoir

(*Le sixième jour*, vv. 699–706)

Du Bartas' technical microcosmic and anatomic knowledge permeates *Le sixième jour*, but he asserts that the poem is a guide for educated readers seeking knowledge about God's masterpiece rather than a manual for doctors and surgeons.[25] Most of his readers had an abiding belief in God's role in the body's creation and in the biblical interpretation of its physical and cognitive forms and functions. In this respect, Du Bartas and Scève shared the same poetic ideals.

The union of man and the world was a basic supposition to Du Bartas. He used a macrocosmic-microcosmic analogy in *Le sixième jour* that assumed that the nature of the body could not be understood without understanding the nature of the universe. His representation of the body was intended to elucidate both the macrocosm and the microcosm. This analogy may appear to the modern mind as a fantastic model of scientific imagination, yet it served him as a meaningful device to clarify anatomy by simple cosmological, geographical and architectural references.

Du Bartas begins mapping the human body, which he designated *la machine humaine* (v. 634) by providing a macroscopic vision of the length, width and depth of its external structures. He compares the eyes, ears, nose, mouth, tongue and teeth to various geographical and architectural features, and then portrays a body metamorphosed into a harmoniously functioning machine. The nose distinguishes odors; the mouth provides a receptive conduit for food; the tongue is a discerning judge; and the teeth serve as a food-processing mill stone (Fig. 1.2., Dryander, woodcut of teeth). Du Bartas demonstrates his familiarity with the functions of the digestive system by describing the metamorphosis of food en route through that system. He views actions within the human body as being analogous to those elsewhere in the cosmos, and mirrors Scève's cosmographic presentation of man as an inverted tree by comparing the body to images of trees which symbolize vast anthropomorphic digestive systems. He describes the alimentary process in *Le sixième jour* as follows:

Le Tout-puissant a fait que la bouche nous rend
Ce que le sein devore, ou que l'aage despend:
Comme les arbres verds par les racines hument
L'humeur qui tient le lieu de l'humeur qu'ils consument.
Dieu la mit en tel lieu, tant afin que le nez
Fit l'essay de l'odeur des vivres destinez
Pour l'humain aliment: qu'afin que nostre veue,
Subtile, discernast l'Anet de la Cigue,
Et du Serpent l'Anguille: ainsi sans faveur

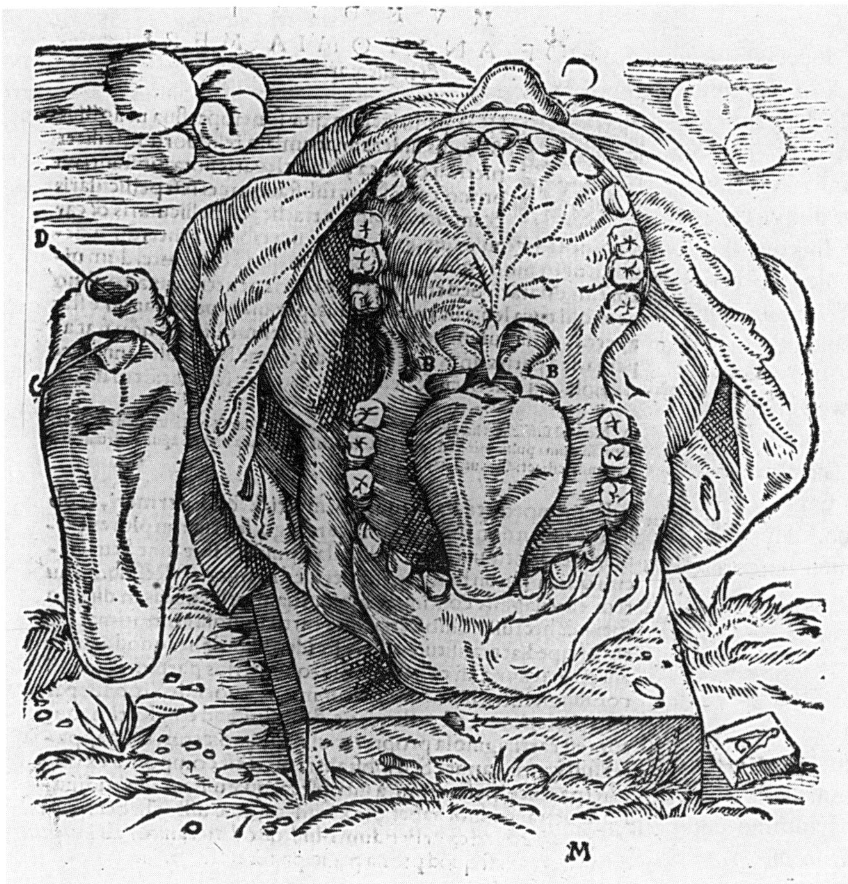

Figure 1.2 Dissection of the mouth, Johann Dryander, woodcut from *Anatomia Mundini*, Marpurgi, In officina Christiani Egenolphi, 1541. (Photo: Courtesy of the National Library of Medicine, Bethesda.)

La langue doit juger de leur vraye saveur.
Un double reng de dens sert à l'ouverture gueule
De forte pallissade: et qui, comme une meule,
Brisant les durs morceaux, envoye promptement
Dans le chaud estomac l'imparfait aliment

(*Le sixième jour*, vv. 555–68)

Succeeding verses analyze alimentation and examine the secret intimacies of the inner parts of the body, with their perplexing designs and intricate labyrinthine paths and structures that serve as organizing images for the ears and brain. The labyrinth symbolizes the sixteenth-century anatomic experience; it reflects how Du Bartas conceived both the world and the body. He reveals his knowledge of the classical image of the labyrinth by linking the one Daedalus designed for King Minos with the divinely-created universe and the divinely-created labyrinths of the *petit monde*.

The labyrinth was intimately involved with Protestantism because it was frequently associated with a pilgrim's passage to Jerusalem[26] (Fig. 1.3., De la Perrière's representation of the labyrinth). Du Bartas may have borrowed this image of the labyrinth as a passageway from Jean Calvin, who used it as a metaphorical structure in his *Institutes*.[27]

Du Bartas begins his corporeal voyage, an anatomically symbolic pilgrimage to the center of the body, through the ears into the eustachian tube. He impressed upon the reader the marvels of the ear's structure, which he considered to be one of the body's most impressive and complex labyrinths.

Mais en quel membre humain luisent plus de merveilles,
. . . . Qu'es conduits tortueux des jumelles oreilles.

(*Le sixième jour*, vv. 597–98)[28]

Movement and intricacy are the two most striking elements in this description; they are also significant factors in Du Bartas' description of the brain. He examines the "cabinets de la double cervelle": the brain's labyrinthine cerebellum and the marvelous Daedalian maze of this *admirable reth*.

Ce Dedale subtil, cest admirable reth
Par les replis duquel l'esprit monte et devale,
Rendant sa faculté vitale, Animale:

(*Le sixième jour*, vv. 654–56)

Du Bartas attempted to place man comfortably in cosmic hierarchies by developing movement in his verse which he illustrated by using the image of the labyrinth. He also used the labyrinth to illustrate his interest in reproducing images of bodily forms and movements. Excellent examples of the body labyrinth analogy are found in his comparison of the ears to

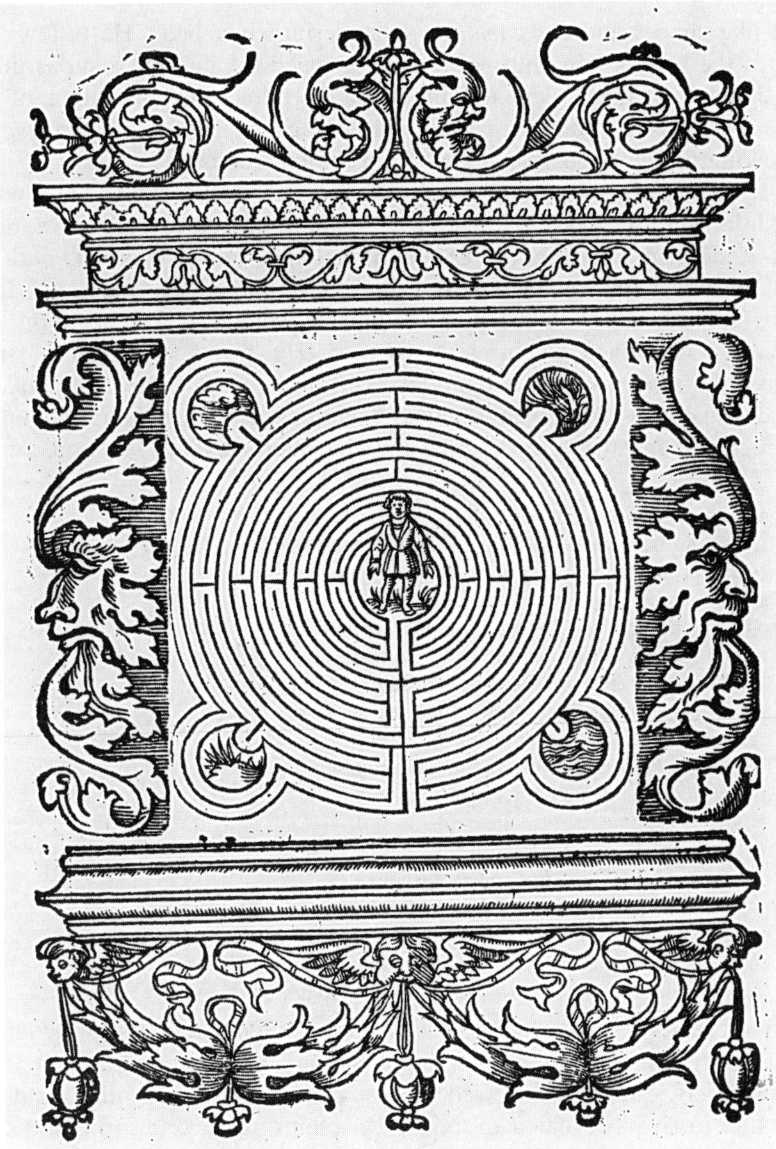

Figure 1.3 Plate of the Labyrinth, Guillaume de la Perrière, from *Le Theatre des Bons Engins*, ca. 1539. (Photo: By Permission of the Folger Shakespeare Library.)

snail-like shapes and ear canals to meandering river beds. He follows the path of the body's labyrinth not simply to reach the interior, such as in the traditional pilgrimage depicted in De la Perrière's representation of the maze, but to view the multiple and perplexing patterns of this *petit monde* by relying on numerous paradigms from the macrocosm.

Just as an excursion into a labyrinth is circuitous, so is Du Bartas' expedition into the body. He uses architectural analogies such as the term *garites*, defined by Cotgrave as "a little lodge for a Sentinell, built on high" (a tower that might represent heaven or something analogous, from where guidance through the maze might be provided). Another term was *limaçons*, snail-like structures, most properly forms which had shells shaped like a *trompe* and a *saquebute* (musical instruments).[29] Finally, he formed analogies from geographical features such as rugged mountains and rocky river valleys to describe the characteristics and functions of the ears.

Le Tout-puissant voulut les oreilles planter
Au haut du bastiment, ainsi qu'en deux garites,
Coquillant leurs canaux, si que les voix conduites
Par les obliques plis de ses deux limaçons
Tousjours de plus en plus en allongeant leurs sons:
Comme l'air de la trompe, ou de la saquebut,
Dure plus que celuy qui passe par la flute:
Ou tout ainsi qu'un bruit s'estend par les destours
D'un escarté valon, ou court avec le cours
D'un fleuve serpentant, ou, rompu, se redouble
Passant entre les dents de quelque roche double.
. . .
Par ce courbé Daedale à l'ésprit nos paroles:
Tout ainsi que le Gers, qui coule, tortueux,
Par le riche Armaignac, n'est tant impetueux
Que la Dou, qui sautant de montaigne en montaigne
Fend d'un cours presque droit de Tarbe la campagne.
(*Le sixième jour*, vv. 604–14, 618–22)

These verses evoke visions of sixteenth-century explorers swept along in the tortuous descents, serpentine bending, and changing channels of French rivers. Du Bartas viewed the ear canals as being similar conduits, their link to rivers revealed in their labyrinthine serpentine form, and convoluted pathways. Du Bartas a compares the journey of air through the ear canals to an echo reverberating across *un escarté valon* following a meandering river bed. Movement into the maze of the brain is also as dangerous and confusing as the exploration of an impetuous river. Its waterways encouraged futile wandering. Yet Du Bartas' verses evoke images of the body's labyrinths in which direct progression is preferred to impetuous exploration. This is particularly illustrated in expressions such as; ''Traversant à droit fil,'' and ''fend d'un cours presque droit.''

The poet realized that the ears and the Dedalian maze of the *rets mirable* were distinguishable from river beds and labyrinths. Nevertheless, they belonged to the same class and were metaphorically interchangeable poetically because they elicited similar responses. Thus, the ears and the cerebellum could replicate river or maze motifs. But more important, to Du Bartas, they became fanciful extensions of meandering or labyrinthine objects in the universe that he could contemplate objectively and depict in the idealized body.

Le sixième jour of *La Première semaine* provides a uniquely poetic picture of the human body. The poem may be distinguished from philosophical and other forms of prose by its stress on pictorial charge, and by the rhythmic power of verse that emphasizes both the body's movements and its structure. Poetry also furnishes a more powerful image of the body than does science, which fails to render an adequately poignant description because it lacks poetry's power to inspire and delight the reader artistically. Du Bartas presents an exuberant poetic and artistic representation of corporeal magnificence, which is a gift of divine glory, to explain the secret workings of the microcosm. Additional elements in the pictorial plan of *La Première semaine*, especially those describing Eve's creation, are examined below (see Quattrocento triangle).

Du Bartas' desire to examine the body's secret inner forms reflects both a scientific and an artistic desire to compose a more lifelike portrait of the body, one blending grace, harmony and proportion. The impact of Renaissance anatomical investigation is evident in the poem, and its presence is undoubtedly due to a combination of factors that relate to Renaissance scientific and religious inquiry. Unquestionably, Renaissance anatomists, who rejected traditional writings on the structure of the body and demanded that it be dissected to gain knowledge of its structure were an enormously important influence. The emergence of Protestantism may also have helped foster the desire to examine the body's inner workings. An examination of this theory, however, which is expounded by Huston Diehl and others, is outside the range of this study.[30] However, both of these views might be considered as motivating factors in the works of Protestant poets such as Du Bartas, and D'Aubigné, whose poem *La Création* is examined next.

3. The Philosopher's Contemplation, Théodore Agrippa D'Aubigné: *La Création* (c. 1623)[31]

D'Aubigné treats man's body cosmographically as a microcosm in much of *La Création*, a poem which he may have intended to be an anatomical text for his son Nathan.[32] He also reflects—at least as much as Du Bartas does—the strong influence of anatomic practices introduced after the publication of Vesalius' treatise. The poet was attracted to the body's physical composition and biological functions, especially its generative capacity and needs for nourishment. (I deal with the anatomical nature of *La Création* in the section below on the poet-prosector.) Most striking of all, however, is D'Aubigné's reflections on the body as a vessel containing the soul, a theme which manifested his preoccupation with philosophical contemplation of the body. In this manner, the poet effects a dualist approach to the body and soul—flesh and spirit—by dividing the poem into fifteen *Chants*, (unlike Du Bartas, who divided his poem into the six days of Creation), each of which inquires into the mysteries of the composition of body and soul.[33]

D'Aubigné incorporated the microcosmic tradition in contemplating the body which he termed *ce petit monde*. He selected the *chef* (head) and the *face* for special study because those parts were not only located where "tout ce qui est celeste" was to be found, but they were what distinguished man from other creatures.

> Une face est en luy differente en figure
> Et separee aussi de toute creature
> . . .
> . . . ce chef s'elevant aux Cieux hauts
> S'estonne en contemplant du monde les merveilles
> Et de son Createur les oeuvres non pareilles.
> Or toute beste jecte en terre son reguard,
> L'ame d'icelle aussi n'a que la terre en part,
> Mais l'home issu du Ciel son oeyle vers luy se tourne.
>
> (*La Création*, *Chant douzième*, 416–17)

Objective truth and knowledge diminish in this poem when D'Aubigné shifts his consideration of the microcosm from the composition of the body to that of the soul, which he asserts categorically is hierarchically superior. He treats the two as distinct entities that Reason can consider separately. Because the body is the soul's shell, and thus its most proximate object, he portrays the soul as the faculty of knowledge that resides in the head. It is capable of contemplating and understanding the attributes of its physical shell but, as we will see, not its own composition.

D'Aubigné relied upon his knowledge of the body's physical structure in a failed attempt to delineate the soul and its structure by transforming its composition and actions into visible entities. But, representing the body's material elements he realized, was far easier than incarnating the soul. He also failed to induce the soul to reveal its own nature and composition; only the Divine Maker could do that. Despite his many poetic talents, D'Aubigné could only speculate on the soul's composition, aware that he lacked the creative capacity to acquire such knowledge. He admitted that "L'Eternel seul le sayt." In the following verses, he and the soul discuss the paradoxical dilemma of its existence and its tangible and intangible nature. He begins the dialogue with the common microcosmic-macrocosmic analogy of the four elements.

Sy des quatre elemans j'estoys creé, allors
Une necessité m'apporteroyt un corps,
Ou que je fusse issue de la semence humaine,
La mort auroyt sur moy puissence souveraine.
Encore moins d'un corps, orres qu'il puisse bien
Engendrer d'autres corps, en moy il ne peut rien:
Je ne fuys engendré, ains de simple nature
Et non comme le corps subject à nourriture.
. . .
Bref je ne sache rien qui seut (rendre) compris
Comment & de quoy sont composez les espris:
C'est chose dificille & qu'on ne peut congnoystre,
L'Eternel seul le sayt, comme auteur de mon estre.

(*La Création*, *Chant douzième*, 435)

The poet's inescapable and ultimate failure to represent materially the soul is illustrated by his use of speculative terms such as *Sy*, *Ou que*, *encore moins*, *Et non comme*, and *Bref.* He finally concludes that these attributes were unknowable to all but the Almighty.

D'Aubigné wanted his work to be as objective as possible, and because the soul was unfathomable he could not long dwell on it because its incorporeality was impossible to depict. Therefore, he devoted the major part of the poem to a description and examination of the body's composition. He even followed anatomists' recommendations to enumerate the bones it contained. Although he revealed the body's physical ambiguities and obscurities, and compared its structure with that of the universe, D'Aubigné remained substantially a poet-observer of the body's structure in order to celebrate God's magnificence, "Combien voyt-on en luy de sagesse profonde / Au bastiment du corps noble, du petit monde!"

4. Alchemical Discourse, François Béroalde de Verville: *Les Cognoissances necessaires* (1583)

Turning to the structures of the universe and the human body as interpreted by the alchemist-philosopher-mathematician-physician François Béroalde de Verville, we find, in his *Les Cognoissances necessaires*, just as in Scève's *Microcosme*, God in the framework of the Creation account. However, there is a great difference in how the two poets analyzed these structures. Astrology and alchemy were then commonly employed in this universal quest, although the considerable influence that the former enjoyed in the Middle Ages was waning. Nevertheless, Scève was much more attracted to astrology and to the zodiacal correspondence between man and the cosmos than to alchemy, although alchemy was still commonly considered to be a valid form of scientific inquiry, an "art which sought to work with nature." According to Lyndy Abraham, "This process required that the alchemist consciously turn back again to the source and origin in order to know the creation and its laws."[34] Doing so required rigorous observation of nature and the use of practical experimental techniques. Béroalde adopted the alchemical approach and ridiculed the astrological.

O grand impieté miserable manie
De chercher nostre sort par une astrologie,
Dont la juste raison qui a jamais ne faut,
Sans descendre icy bas est demeuree en haut.
Cassés, brisés, rompés ces estranges mesures
Destruisés mesprisés ces menteuses figures,

(*Les Cognoissances*, f. 5v)

Alchemical language was central to Béroalde's spiritual and poetic thought; he used it as a code in his account of Creation to decipher the microcosmic-macrocosmic analogy between the universe and the human body.[35] He also used it to create a correspondence between the structures of the universe and of man, merging them into harmonious and ordered wholes. Béroalde resembles several of his contemporaries, e.g., Scève, Du Bartas and D'Aubigné, in explaining his motivation for writing the poem and his objectives in studying "ce petit monde hoste de l'univers."[36]

Je recherche de tout la forme interieure,
La matiere du monde & de ce qui demeure,
Dessous l'enclos du ciel, & les justes accords,
Qui tiennent les espris arrestés à leurs corps,
. . .
Je cherche tels secres sans peine & sans envie,
Et aux opinions n'estant point arresté,
De nature je dis selon la verité.

(*Les Cognoissances*, f. 1v)

But unlike those poets, Béroalde's aim was not didactic, and he made few stylistic concessions to his readers.[37] His purpose was simply to pay homage to ''Monsieur P. de l'estoille conseilleur du Roy, & audiencier à la chancellerie de Paris'' in order to ''recognoistre par quelque bon service les biens que vous m'avés faits.''[38]

The basic difference between *Les Cognoissances* and the poems of Du Bartas and D'Aubigné is that Béroalde does not describe the body in encyclopedic fashion or even allude to an anatomical investigation which might contribute to the poem's scientific appeal. Furthermore, he does not divide the poem into ''Jours'' or ''Chants'' to order the days or events of Creation as Du Bartas and D'Aubigné did. Instead, *Les Cognoissances* is characterized by the lack of an organizing plan and abstract and non-pictorial elements. The poem describes the states of the universe and the human body as they were being formed, in which the points of reference combine two different accounts. The creation myth is one, with God depicted as the author, or architect. The other integrates alchemical theories and Hermetic philosophy, with which Béroalde sought to interpret the divine scheme of things, considering God and an invisible world, but which he hoped to make visual by his description.

The long portrayal of the creation of the world in *Les Cognoissances* is interesting primarily because it illustrates what the poet thought about alchemical transmutation. Béroalde's account prepares the reader to interpret the pre-physical form of the body and to examine the process of its formation as well as its place in the macrocosmic-microcosmic structure. *Les Cognoissances* links God, man and matter inseparably in one marvelous design. God's handiwork encompasses all of nature; everything is modeled and nourished by His light or fire which continuously flows from heaven to earth.

> Certes comme Dieu est d'infini puissance,
> Sa grandeur passe aussi toute force & science,
> Et ne peut on trouver tant cét abisme est creux,
> L'estat de la raison de ses faicts merveilleux.
> Car de rien il tira toute la secheresse,
> Du plus gros element qui au plus bas se baisse,
> Dessous toute l'humeur, que d'une mesme sujet
> Il a fait eschapper comme l'air qu'il ha fait,
> Et le feu nourrissant toutes choses crees,
> Ayant fait en un coup tant d'essences meslees:

(*Les Cognoissances*, f. 2v)

Les Cognoissances contains the customary eulogy to God and His infinite powers, after which the poet examines the ''Creation de la premiere matiere'' and the universe as a formless void whose chaotic elements are gradually structured through the medium of His strength.

> Tirant de ce Chaos où la matiere infuse,
> Estoit infiniment confuse non confuse,
> Les quatre qualité, & premiers elemens
> Qui sont de ce qui est forces commencements
> . . .
>
> (*Les Cognoissances*, f. 2r)

Béroalde expands this image of the four elements in subsequent verses, which are intended to praise particular manifestations of the workings of God, especially the creative power of His voice. Thus, the forms of life are spoken into existence (following Genesis).

> Or le Dieu tout puissant . . .
> . . .
> Crea cét existant dont son juste parler
> Tira les cieux, le feu, la mer, la terre, l'air,
> Faisant ce monde entier d'une belle mesure,
> Durant six jours certains & non par avanture.
> . . .
> Il crea univers par sa vertu divine.
>
> (*Les Cognoissances*, f. 3r-v)

The poet assumed that God created the ''first matter,'' which was no particular thing but yet everything. This matter linked the divinely-created terrestrial and celestial worlds.

> Dieu tout sage & tout fort de soy mesme arracha
> La force, & la vertu, qu'au monde il attacha,
> Et de ce qui est rien à nostre cognoissance,
> Fit de cét univers l'universelle essence,
> . . .
> Le ciel qui n'est rien qu'eau, fut l'essence premiere,
> La terre fut apres, qui d'une autre matiere
> Contraire & non contraire, & en soy s'amassant,
> Alloit vers le millieu peu à peu s'abaissant.
>
> (*Les Cognoissances*, f. 9v)

Béroalde believed that he was furthering God's work by attempting to ''peindre exactement cette essence creee.''[39] Phraseology such as *meslange*, *chaos obscur*, *part à part*, and *sous les lois de ton art* suggests an alchemical art. His use of words that combine alchemy and an artistic code add to the beauty of his verses.

Arrestons nous un peu, & parmi ce meslange
Gardons qu'en ce discours, ce tout cy ne se change
En un chaos obscur, mais prenant part à part
Taschons si nous pouvons sous les lois de ton art,
De peindre exactement cette essence creee,
Comme Dieu l'ordonna la premiere journee.

(*Les Cognoissances*, f. 9v)

Béroalde also seems to implicate an alchemical phenomenon in the generation of the human body. His preoccupation with alchemical terminology (e.g. sulphur, mercury, salt and vitriol) to denote entities in the macrocosmic world as well as in man the microcosm forms part of his erudite allusion to hermetic information. However, he neither analyzes nor explains the meaning of the various elements and alchemical processes, nor the lessons to be derived therefrom. He leaves this largely for the reader to puzzle out, although it was probably readily comprehensible to most well-informed sixteenth-century readers.

The following verses illustrate Béroalde's use of alchemical structures and images to depict the elements in the universe that were available for use in the generation of the body.

Le soufre, & le salpetre & le transporte aux cieux[40]
Qui pressés par le vent degoutent sur la terre
La neige, le frimas, la gresle, le tonnerre:
Car il mesle là haut, ce qui y est porté,
En tout corps et en l'air par la force agité.

(*Les Cognoissances*, f. 11v)

Thus it was possible for the universe (the great world) to serve as a prototype for man (the little world). But Béroalde concedes that man was created "in the image of God."

L'homme portast en soy, plus juste et plus parfait,
Les traits plus accomplis de son sacre pourtrait.

(*Les Cognoissances*, f. 12r)

Amid the hermetic information that he divulges, however, Béroalde reminds the reader that his primary interest is in his poetic art. He illustrates the generation of man from elements in the mineral kingdom, yet incorporates some clearly explanatory verses, as if to steer a middle course between alchemy, represented below by the term *foudre*, and the divine plan, perhaps in order to avoid becoming alienated from God.

Muse arrestons un peu, que le foudre n'estonne
Cét homme que voicy, que le grand Dieu façonne,
Et devant qu'assembler tant de sujets divers,
Voyons ce petit monde hoste de l'univers.

(*Les Cognoissances*, f. 11v)

The poet then introduces additional alchemical terms that he integrates with the divine role in the generation of the human body. He pays particular attention to the actions of the hands of God, yet within the context of the imagery in these verses he might well have been suggesting that specific alchemical processes were involved (e.g., *croistre & changer*, *feu secret*, *s'eschaufer*, *moulant*, *transforma en une autre substance*).

> Adonq il prit la terre & d'une main heureuse,
> A lieu que paravant elle estoit otieuse,
> La trempant en l'humeur, la fit croistre & changer,
> Et par son feu secret justement s'eschaufer,
> Puis la moulant aux traits de sa sainte semblance,
> Sa masse il transforma en une autre substance,
> Luy Dieu qui avoit fait de rien ce grand enclos,
> Fit de la poudre chair, sang, peau, veines, & os,
>
> (*Les Cognoissances*, f. 12r)

The undifferentiated earth has been dissolved by a process known as *dissolutio* or *solve* to form *vaine argile* (f. 5v), the basic building material.[41] This was the generally accepted first step in the alchemical process, which was a seemingly backward one that required the destruction or dissolution of an old form to reconstitute the new. The body of man is generated out of this newly created pure form, which was known as the *coagula*, or transformation, as it was taking shape.

Béroalde continues to focus on the handiwork of God in the next section of the poem, which sets the tone admirably for the remainder of the work. These verses, which concentrate on love, the characterization of woman, and the harmony and perfection of her body, begin by portraying man's body as being

> . . . formé d'une juste harmonie
> Eut la perfection par l'effait de sa vie.
> Mais cét homme est tout seul & la derniere main,
> De Dieu n'a pas encore parfait le genre humain.
>
> (*Les Cognoissances*, f. 13v)

The poet provides only meager anatomical information about the male body; it is limited to enumerations such as "chair, sang, peau, veines & os" and the statement that God endowed him with "deux pieds, il luy donna les yeux, / Au plus haut de son chef pour regarder les cieux" (f. 12r).

The parts of the anatomy that Béroalde lists are common to all, and thus neither specifically male nor female. However, he is more attentive to the presentation of the female body, which he describes by using a curious amalgam of considerations of her anatomy and her biblical and contemporary social identities. Adhering to Genesis 2:24, Béroalde asserts that woman was created to console man and to relieve his loneliness. He stresses her role as pacifier and peacemaker.

A qui peut il conter ce qu'il a dedans l'ame,
S'il est seul eslongné, d'une benigne femme,
. . .
D'une femme qui peut tant est ingenieuse,
Transformer le malheur, en une vie heureuse,
Et par ses doux attraits tous forceans, tous divins,
Des hommes adoucir les contraires destins,

(*Les Cognoissances*, f. 14r)

These verses depict woman as one in whom the elements live at peace, a pleasingly proportioned divine creation in which harmony reigned. Béroalde represents her in a manner consistent with conventional iconography as "toute amour, toute grace" (f. 14r) rather than strictly as a manifestation of the elements in the cosmos. Predictably, in considering the poet's physical description of "la personne seconde," Eve, "cette femme encore toute nouvelle / Delicate, amoureuse, en forme toute belle," (f. 15r) we learn little of her physical makeup except that she is formed from "la matiere seconde." Otherwise, Béroalde is largely faithful to the biblical source. She is "Os venus de ses os, sang venu de son sang, / chair de sa propre chair tiree de son flang" (f. 15r).

Béroalde does not display the explicit misogyny found in D'Aubigné's *La Création*, although he does include misogynist commonplaces such as the pernicious power of woman (see below). Yet the abuse that he directs at her seems to be intended to denigrate her social identity rather than her body. We discover slightly more about her if we apply the poet's information to the iconography of contemporary woman or to femininity in general. For example, there is a striking example of Béroalde's notion of woman and the unparalleled "pouvoir de la femme" in verses which refer to her hard and deceitful nature, to her "feminine wiles," and to the male victims who have lost their hearts to these deceptions.

Si discrette elle veut usant de sa douceur
Eteindre les rigueurs qu'elle couve en son coeur.
. . .
La femme n'y est point, ou n'est encores veue
Donq' sa puissance aussi ne sera point cognue.
Si rien à desirer ne se trouvoit icy,
De desirs nous n'aurions jamais le coeur saisi,
Et l'amour non amour n'useroit à outrance,
De ses aveugles traits sur nos coeurs sans deffence,

(*Les Cognoissances*, f. 14r)

On the whole, however, while providing little anatomical information or microcosmic comparisons, the poem displays a certain awareness of woman's role in Creation, and her character.

The remaining verses of the *Les cognoissances* evolve into an exaltation of chastity, a condemnation of the dangers of female sexuality, and the importance of marriage, "le dernier but des chastes passions," (f. 20v). These are all familiar positions of the patriarchal construction of feminine nature developed by Béroalde.

It is interesting to note that the poet provides a final glimpse of the *petit monde* which he links with the theme of marriage. He declares:

Je ne suis pas asses pour chanter dignement
Cet estat bien heureux où du commencement
Nos ancestres rangés, & faits maistres du monde
Furent d'un petit monde une forme seconde.
Or le monde se dit pour autant qu'il est net,
Et ce petit ausi pource qu'il est parfet,
Et qu'en cette union l'honnesteté gardee
Fait croistre le vouloir dessus la chose aymee.
Le mariage aussi commence par destin,
Se forme par amour, par honneur prend la fin:
Car nulle n'est jamais à sa moitié donnee,
Si tout premier au ciel elle n'est ordonner,

(*Les Cognoissances*, f. 20v)

The poem finishes on an hermetical note, its final verses form a discourse on the secrets of the "Le Mercure des Philosophes" and culminate with a dedication of the body to God.

The representation of the body in *Les Cognoissances necessaires* is ambiguously dualistic because, as previously noted, it develops from two fundamental powers: the creation myth (with God the architect) and the alchemical process (with which the poet constructs the cosmos symbolically). Béroalde fully developed the two representations.

5. Poet-Physician, Joseph Du Chesne, Sieur de la Violette: *L'anatomie du petit monde* (1584)

Moving from Hermetic philosophy and alchemy to medicine and physiology, one is attracted to the descriptive and interpretative poem *L'Anatomie du petit monde* by the Protestant poet-physician-diplomat Joseph Du Chesne. *L'Anatomie* appears initially to be important to this study and to the representation of the body as a microcosm because of its title, Du Chesne's medical training, and the light the poem might cast on sixteenth-century anatomical studies.[42] But while the poem provides an interesting anatomical representation of the body (see below), it fails to treat the Creation or provide an extended analysis of the body as a microcosm. Rather, the poem's importance is found in moral and ethical discourses that interpret the body after the Adamic Fall as being the site of debilitating and corrupting passions that test the soul's constancy. Absent is the stress on the harmony of the composition of the body found in Béroalde de Verville, Du Bartas and D'Aubigné. Du Chesne's model of the body depicts its imbalances and imperfections rather than the qualities of perfection that generally provided his contemporaries with standards of measurement for the universe and the body. He announces in the *pièces limnaires* (''dedicatory pieces'') that he has

> composé une petite Anatomie spirituelle de l'homme, en laquelle je declare l'usage depravé des parties de ceste creature la plus accomplie de toutes avant le peché, & maintenant la plus corrompue & miserable depuis sa rebellion.[43]

Du Chesne provides a didactic approach to examining the body that developed from a perspective of ''l'usage des parties.'' By insisting upon employing this perspective, his approach differed significantly from other Creation poets who studied and praised the actions and effects of bodily organs for the ''pleasure and content'' of their inexperienced readers. *L'Anatomie* was also directed at a specific reader.

> O homme qui ne sais quel est le vrai usage
> Des parties du corps bien agencé,
> Li-moi ce beau discours par du Chesne tracé:
> Et lors l'ayant apris tu en seras plus sage.

The poem is fairly short compared to Béroalde's *Les Cognoissances*, D'Aubigné's *La Création*, and far shorter than the encyclopedic work of Du Bartas. It consists of fifty *huitains* (400 lines) followed by twelve sonnets on human vices. These include several topics relating to the representation of the body; e.g., *l'avarice*, *la paillardise*, *la prodigalité*, and *la paresse*. The work contains obvious macrocosmic-microcosmic implications. Du Chesne's approach to studying the body in terms of what constitutes the microcosm is represented in terms of his focus on related vices. This is apparent in the following verses in which the body is depicted in each line as being composed of the four elements. Yet each line is completed by references to negative attributes: vices and diseases. Instead of glorifying the body as a microcosm, Du Chesne vilifies its substance. Rather than acclaiming the marvels achieved by the Divine Maker in the structure and composition of the body, *L'Anatomie* expounds on its corruption.

> Dedans un petit corps qui veut voir tout le Monde,
> Le feu dedans un coeur, tout bouïllant de fureur,
> La terre dans des os, l'apui de tout malheur

Dedans l'humide sang, l'inconstance de l'onde,
Et l'air dans des poulmons rien que peste souflans,
Jette l'oeil sur mes vers l'homme anatomizans:
L'homme un monde petit, ou du grand on peut lire
Le foible apui, la peste, & l'inconstance, & l'ire.

(*L'Anatomie*, *Huitain* I)

Du Chesne's view of man as microcosm was the setting for his interpretation of the aftermath of the Fall, a ground upon which he propagandized and aired bitter resentment over the religious wars, and a vehicle of satire. He propounded the idea that man's place in the universe was different from that of any other animal, "une figure / La plus admirable en nature," (Huitain XVIII). Yet, in another huitain Du Chesne displayed distinct anti courtier satire and emphasized the imperfections and disharmony of man's body, a fact that man tried ineffectively to hide by using exotic fragrances and embellishments. He satirizes the beauty practices of the courtier, whose sole aim is to remain attractive to the opposite sex.

Parfume toi ô homme Dameret[44]
Cent fois le jour des odeurs sabeenes,
Embaume-toi des liqueurs indienes
Tu ne rendras pourtant ton corps plus net,
Ta nature est tellement imparfaite
Pleine d'ordure & de corruption,
Que tu pourrois au lieu de sentir bon
Empunaisir & l'ambre & la civette.

(*L'Anatomie*, Huitain XXXV)

Du Chesne's fundamental purpose in his work was to expose the irony of the vain arrogance of man who, in attempting to elevate himself on the Chain of Being, knew that the body would ultimately be reduced by death, the great leveler, into "une charongne puante" (Huitain II).

This has been a wide-ranging study, examining a variety of ways in which the representation of the human body as a microcosm was approached within the framework of the Creation myth in Renaissance poetry. While several poems exhibit a discernible and logical development within the genre of Creation poems, others diverge significantly from that narrative structure. These poems are stylistically very different and vary in length and quality, reflecting the poets' artistic abilities, interests and preoccupations. Yet each poem is a fascinating study of the human body, and collectively they illustrate the various ways that Renaissance Creation poets sought to represent it.

The representation of the body by Creation poets was marked by the process through which they aspired, using a microcosmic theory descended from Pythagoras, a theological framework; paraphrase of the Book of

Genesis, and poetic metaphors, to represent man as the crowning achievement of creation. As we have shown, most of these poets adhered to microcosmic theories. Yet, they described the human body by means of microcosm-macrocosm analogies combined with various disciplines, i.e., alchemy, astrology, cosmography (geography), music, architecture, medicine and art, thereby transmuting disorder into order. They portrayed the body and soul together as the quintessence of life.

Some poets, in their desire to understand the structures of the cosmos and man, found relationships between the shape of the body and the empirical mapping of terrestrial regions. Others created parallels between anatomy and alchemy to demonstrate that man and his world were composed of the same elements. Each poet had a distinctive way of describing the body, generally by reducing its universe to visual terms and producing declarations glorifying this microcosm's marvelous organic composition. Their purpose in studying the body as a microcosm was to describe and gain knowledge of man, the central and most important element in the universe. They also aspired to praise God and to "please and content" their readers while instructing them.

As the Renaissance progressed, attempts to unify and understand man's fragmented being became evermore extreme. Predictibly, then, we find that Renaissance figures such as Montaigne began to criticize the efforts by some to depict and thereby understand man's structure through microcosmic theories. These critics believed that the ancient opinion that man was a microcosmic model of the universe had been fantastically strained by the idea that there were certain correspondences and parallels between man's body and the great variety of things extant in the universe such as stars, plants, and minerals. As Montaigne observed, despite examining man from all possible macrocosmic-microcosmic correspondences, it was impossible to grasp his nature. What is implicit in Montaigne's writing and notable in the poetry of Du Bartas and Du Chesne is the trend away from viewing man solely in terms of the microcosmic analogy, and the belief that empirical methods should be employed in the study of the human body. But above all, it is the acceptance and use of anatomy, a science that demanded opening this little world in order to reveal its secrets, that marks a transition stage in the history of microcosmic theories. Prosecting the body opened it to the authority of the scientist's gaze and to the art of the poet, allowing them to more thoroughly view the anatomic marvels—the birth, growth and decay—of this "machine of the universe."

Anatomical Inquiry:
The Poet-prosector and the post-mortem

> Anatomie donc, selon son étymologie, est une entiere et parfaite division ou resolution artificielle du corps humain en ses parties, tant universelles que particulieres, simples que composées.
>
> (Paré, *De l'Anatomie*, Livre I, 108)

Human anatomies, which were practiced more widely during the Renaissance than ever before, acquired expanded new dimensions through attempts to gain a better understanding of the body by exploring both the organic world and the soul that lay within its sheltering sphere.

Andreas Vesalius (1514–1564), whose famous *De humani corporis fabrica* (1543) and *Epitome* (1543) describe and illustrate the dissection and physical examination of a human body, was "the first modern anatomist to place his study on a firm foundation of observation."[45] He lamented man's disregard for self-knowledge and reproached physicians who failed to examine physically the body's structure. It was inappropriate, he wrote,

> . . . that in the pursuit of studies so varied, . . . that man be completely unknown to himself; and that the structure of instruments so divinely created by the Great Artificer of all things should remain unexamined: . . .[46]

Following Vesalius, another renowned Renaissance physician, Ambroise Paré (1517–90), provided continued impetus for this movement by relating in his surgical treatises how sixteenth century man speculated upon bewildering phenomena such as the heavens and the dimensions of the earth. He chastised his contemporaries for their disinterest in examining the body's anatomical structure to discover its "excellence et merveilleuse composition" and thereby to acquire self-knowledge in so doing.[47]

Paré, who blended Classical, Medieval and Renaissance medical theories in his work, affirmed that anatomical science was a "chose digne d'estre cognuë par tout homme de bon esprit."[48] He advocated close visual scrutiny of the body because "Les Elemens de nostre corps sont les parties solides et similaires, . . . qui sont faciles à cognoistre, à cause qu'ils se representent au sens de la veuë." [49] Vesalius and Paré recommended abandoning a reliance on conjecture and adopting instead precise, fully-documented investigative techniques to achieve the goal of self-knowledge. They advised anatomists to begin the exploration of the body by empirical observation, and to conform to a descriptive plan to produce a dissection-based anatomy that furnished "histories" or descriptions of the individual organs and parts of the body. This commentary should be methodically arranged *a capite ad calcem* (the head-to-toe order of classical origin),[50] proceeding (according to Paré) from the universal ("Teste, Thorax, Ventre") to the particular ("comme les parties d'icelles"), and from the simple to the more complex.[51]

These and similar recommendations by Paré, Vesalius and other Renaissance anatomists not only inspired more frequent and more scientific anatomical inquiry, but they also attracted poets to the subject because it furthered their search for self-knowledge and their desire to promote the new poetic genres of scientific poetry and encyclopedism. This is illustrated by the many poems devoted to the body.

Little scholarly research has been done on the anatomical examination of man's body as treated in sixteenth century poetry. This section is intended to fill this void at least partially by focusing specifically on prosection in the works of Guillaume De Saluste Sieur Du Bartas, Théodore Agrippa D'Aubigné, and Joseph Du Chesne.[52] Each pursued scientific inquiries reflecting existing knowledge and contemporary concerns for performing anatomies, and each rationalized them poetically.

I examine the empirical approaches these poets took to the external and internal anatomical representations of the body, to their representations of idealized forms of the body, and to the relationship they sought between language and truth to depict the body using a scientific discipline. Each of these poets, for whom the search for truth was fundamental, had distinct goals and applied a particular poetic strategy in exploring and anatomizing the human body in verse. They intended to praise God as the architect of man's structure, but they had more substantial objectives, i.e., to understand man anatomically, to reveal the secrets of his physical structure, to understand human diseases and remedies, to uncover the significance of man's role in the visible universe, and to present their findings scrupulously. These aspirations, united with an awareness of their poetic capabilities, were often proclaimed in appeals to the Muse or to God for inspiration. The following material represents three distinct poetic approaches to the anatomical examination of man's body.

1. Théodore Agrippa D'Aubigné, *La Création*: Anatomical Contemplation

D'Aubigné assumed the mantle of an ideal observational anatomist to anatomize the body elaborately in *La Création*, and to provide "histories," descriptions and surveys of the body's parts and organs. The final third of his poem is composed of a series of physiological observations divided into five cantos (*Chants*, 11–15) that contain an internal arrangement inspired by the traditional head-to-toe order. The anatomy of the body is condensed into the first three, the soul and its movements into the last two.

D'Aubigné separated his anatomical teaching into three phases, each of which formed a compendium of the contents of the *Epitome's* six books. These were a) Thoracic Viscera, Abdominal Viscera and Organs of Reproduction; b) the Brain and Nervous System; and c) Bones, Cartilages, Muscles, Ligaments, and the Vascular System.[53] Although the order of the anatomical teaching in the cantos differs from that found in the *Epitome*, D'Aubigné obviously appropriated much of his anatomical material from Vesalius' work; he repeatedly paraphrased the Vesalian text poetically. This is especially evident in his enumeration of the parts of the body. His interpretation of the seven pairs of cranial nerves is an excellent example.[54] The poet renders the discursive Vesalian description of those nerves as follows (I have cited just four of them because the Vesalian text is lengthy and the four adequately illustrate the point.):

Le premier donne voye à l'esprit qui faict voir,
  Le seconde distribue aux muscles le mouvoir
  Des yeux, & par le tiers la narine aprestee
  A sentir toute chose à elle presantee.
Outre il sort un rameau de luy, dict gustatif,
  De la langue mobille un vray preparatif
  A gouster toute chose, & le quart couple mande
  Au palays mesme effect qu'à la langue friande.

(*La Création, Chant douzième*, 415–16)

D'Aubigné was also influenced by anatomists other than Vesalius, notably Paré, from whom he borrowed superficial expressions associated with the first cranial nerves such as "l'esprit visuel." This was particularly evident in vocabulary associated with the skull and brain, such as Paré's comparison of the skull to a rampart and his references to the "temperament" of the brain.

Ce siege de rayson, membre pituyteux,
  Mol & froyt de son estre est divisé en deux,
. . .
Ce crane doncques est comme un rempar trés fort

(*La Création, Chant douzième*, 412–13)

Paré's elaborate descriptions (which are less technical than Vesalius') are represented as follows. The cranium (designated by *Teste*) "est le siege des sens, et rempart de raison."[55] "La superficie exterieure du cerveau est molle", and the brain's "temperament [is] froid et humide."[56]

In subsequent verses of *La Création*, D'Aubigné uses poetic latitude in describing the brain to create captivating images of the *avare amasseur* and the ideal composition of the cranium.[57]

Nature a faict ainsi que l'avare amasseur
Lequel, pour conserver & cacher en lieu seur
Son tresor precieux, il cherche lieu duysible,
Sur tout secret & fort, & le moins acessible.
(*La Création, Chant douzième*, 413)

D'Aubigné clearly considered his role to be that of an observer describing the body's external and internal features rather than that of a poet prosector who actually performed dissections. He did not explain why he undertook such a rigorous textbook anatomical examination, yet he did reveal its divine purpose when he began to examine the *chef d'oeuvre exquis* of the *grand Architecte*.[58] He started by viewing the body as an assemblage of *membres* and enumerated its individual parts (''la teste, epaulles, bras & mains, / Les cuisses, jambes, piez,'') before focusing on the thorax (''le col, costes & reins'' [p.406]). Then, using *offices* as his criteria he elaborates on the functions of the body and the hierarchy existing among its parts.[58]

Car rien ne se peut voir en ce chef d'oeuvre exquis
Qui n'y soyt agencé ainsi qu'il est requis.
Plusieurs membres y sont aptes à son service
Lesquelz tous d'un acord exercent leur office.
Que si quelq'un d'entr' eux on desire offencer,
L'autre membre survient pour le mal devencer;
La mutuelle peur q'un d'eux soufre moleste
Faict pour le guarantir emouvoir tout le reste.
(*La Création, Chant unzieme*, 405–6)

D'Aubigné also interpreted the body as being a metaphor for the structure of society. He used social terminology to illustrate that its parts and organs (*membres*) were linked in alliances of solidarity and sympathy.[60] Accordingly, there were three noble organs in the thorax that ruled over the others, to which D'Aubigné added a fourth, *les testiculles* (discussed below under gender).

Troys choses sont au corps dont le reste despend,
C'est à savoir le foye origine du sang,
Le coeur & le cerveau, parties principales
Et le vray entretien des essences vitalles.
On en peut dire quatre à bon droyt, car du corps
Ce n'est rien ou bien peu, les testiculles hors:
(*La Création, Chant unzieme*, 406)

D'Aubigné gives little indication of an actual dissection in *La Création*. However, his poem *La Sorcière*, written earlier, might be considered a precursor although it did not treat the Creation, because it gave considerable scope to a post-mortem examination. He even included himself in a group of prosectors of a suspected witch, declaring that ''nous facions . . . la vraie anatomie.'' He echoed the scientific curiosity (''Pour congnoistre'') associated with medical dissections and provided a rationale for beginning the procedure.

Elle est morte, c'est fait, que de mon ennemie
Nous facions à ce coup la vraie anatomie,
Pour congnoistre commant, sans lui avoir fait tort,
Aux causes de la vie elle a senty la mort.

(*La Sorcière*, vv. 67–70)[61]

Contemplation (''Contemplon donc cest home en sa creation'' [p. 402]) provided D'Aubigné with a basic metaphor for observing and interpreting the body. He considered it to be one of the four Cardinal Virtues possessed by the *cerveau & chef* (''De ses quatre vertus qu'on nomme cardinales: / La premiere consiste en contenplation [sic]''), and linked it to the function of the eyes to provide a visual means of comprehending his subject.

Par les yeux l'home peut mainte affaire ordonner,
Par les yeux on luy voyt la chose discerner,
Par les yeux il admire, reguarde & contemple
Le total espendu au dedans du Ciel emple.

(*La Création, Chant douzième*, 418)

In any case, while the poem reveals his medical interest, the body is presented in the form of a contemplation or a meditation which is meant to be illustrative or explanatory, and therefore of didactic intent. Rather than displaying a body in a anatomy theater, D'Aubigné seems to be referring to anatomical illustrations and medical treatises. *La Création* has strong visual appeal, yet the poet struggles with the problems of poetic representations of the body and, especially, of the soul (which is examined below). He served as demonstrator, observer and commentator rather than prosector, and used his considerable visual and tactile experience, combined with meditative adoration of the intricacies of the anatomy, in exploring the body. Beauty, D'Aubigné implied, is beheld by the eyes; this may be applied unequivocally to his visual evaluation of the body.

L'home privé des yeux a bien peu de plaisir:
Le beau entre le laid il ne peut pas choisir,
Il est forclos des ars & de la jouissance:
Bref c'est un corps sans corps, confiné & reduyt

(*La Création, Chant douzième*, 419)

D'Aubigné's use of words such as *voyr*, *observer*, *lignes*, *traiz*, and *tableau* demonstrates that he was fully conversant with artistic and architectural terminology and had adopted the current vogue of linking painting to poetry. He depicted the body as God's masterpiece, which could be best comprehended through a visual medium that offered structural equivalents and architectural constructs.

> Ce corps fust excellant sur toute creature
> . . .
> Et d'art ingenieux divinement hanté.
> Tant en lignes que traiz, là le grand Architecte
> Batissant ceste ouvrage ouvrier se manifeste,
> (*La Création*, *Chant unzième*, 405)

Although he began by expressing his admiration for the architectural and artistic design of the body, D'Aubigné later concentrated more on its bewildering complexity, and the fact that verbal description and tactile experience could not embrace the totality of the body, much less that of the soul.

> On peut voyr comme un corps touscher ne sauroyt pas
> Un corps en son total. . .
> (*La Création*, *Chant quinzième*, 438)

D'Aubigné described the marvels of the human body throughout *La Création*. He mastered a systematic and thorough study of it and responded successfully to contemporary anatomical practices, carefully implementing the recommendations of renowned Renaissance scholars and physicians. He thereby provided not only a methodical approach to a complete and perfect knowledge of the body, but a poetic insight into its realities.

However, as revealed in the final two cantos, the fundamental didactic purpose of *La Création* may have been as much a quest for self-knowledge (by anatomically describing the human body) as it was an effort to discern or create a soul that is fixed, tangible and knowable. D'Aubigné struggled to shape a satisfactory visual representation of the soul which was, artistically speaking, more challenging and difficult than representing the body. He was aware of his inability to express the inward nature of both the spirit and the soul without an outward and bodily demonstration. His description is couched in terms that expose awareness of his poetic limitations.

> Or doncques il me fault chanter à mon pouvoir
> Les effects merveilleux que l'ame peut avoir.
> Dispose toy, ma plume, ores que soys petite,
> Pour ce divin subjet traicter comme il merite.
> Muse divine, vien, vien me donner secours,
> Puis que faire me faut de l'ame emple discours,
> Vien Muse, je te pry, qui de bien dire as grace,
> Afin qu'heureusement & à mon gré le face.

(*La Création*, *Chant quatorzième*, 431)

D'Aubigné's emphasis on corporality, the priority of sight and, especially, the medium of painting, provided him with a motif for expressing the nature of both the soul and the spirit. He shaped his view of the soul, and hopefully that of the reader, by using genres such as painting and portraiture, thus frequently using visual vocabulary. The terms *voir* and *contempler des yeux*, which are used to describe the body, are repeated in *Chant quatorzième* and in the beginning of *Chant quinzième*, where he combines them with pictorial images to frame his subject. Indeed, D'Aubigné asserted that the soul, unlike the body, was knowable only to God "C'est chose dificille & qu'on ne peut congnoystre, / L'Eternel seul le sayt, comme auteur de mon estre" (435). However, he began by envisioning the soul because he considered its further exploration necessary. He then introduces the poetic *je*, into the poem, thereby involving himself intimately in the inquiry, and expressing apprehension about the adequacy of his poetic talents for describing a *divine essence* that is "invisible à tous corporelz yeux" (433). Yet, D'Aubigné devises a poetic way to "see" the soul by means of a dialogue with it.

May ozeroys je bien faire cela sans toy,
  Ame, unique vigueur de ce qui vit en moy?
  Seroys je tant hardy d'entrer en la cariere
  Et que par un mespris je te laissasse ariere?
Rien moins, mays tant s'en faut que j'entreprene rien
  Sans toy, ame celeste, où gist mon plus grand bien!
  Aproche-toy de moy, ame tant excellante,
  Puis que l'ocasion à mes yeux se presante.

(*La Création*, *Chant quatorzième*, 432)

Thus invited to the discourse, the soul locates itself "Dans le corps des humains, temple du trés haut Dieu," where it is placed as a painting with *ligne & trayt* that must be closely observed and contemplated to gain further understanding. Throughout the following verses, then, the soul teaches the poet and his readers how to behold.

Or sy plus emplement tu desire savoir
  Mes vertueux effectz, il t'est besoign de voir
  Un tableau de grand pris où mon ymage est peinte,
  Mis au temple de Dieu comme chose trés sainte
Iceluy t'aprendra en le contemplant bien
  Tout ce qui est en moy d'excellant et de bien.
  Pren y guarde de prés, voy le bien & observe
  Chacune ligne & trayt, rien n'est là qui ne serve.

(*La Création*, *Chant quatorzième*, 435)

Skeptically, and in a move which perhaps indicated that he considered this art to be an illusion, D'Aubigné interrupted the soul's discourse to "see" this miraculous *tableau* for himself, hoping that it would help him with the remainder of his poetic discourse.

Voulant voir quel il est (l'interrompu discours
De l'ame) incontinant j'euz au tableau recours,
Soubz espoir par le voir mieux discourir le reste,
D'autant que le subject n'estoyt là manifeste.
Entré que fus au temple, incontinant je voy
Ce tableau tant exquis, oeuvre digne de foy,
De tel qu'on y voyt de l'ame un vray indice.
(*La Création, Chant quatorzième*, 435)

While still in the temple cum art gallery, D'Aubigné declared "Je me trensporte voir l'autre costé du temple. / Là je voy l'esprit faict à l'image de Dieu" (437). His efforts to describe materially the spirit are replete with the same ineffable and perplexing circularities that he used to deduce the material nature of the soul. Corporeal vocabulary again provided the standard of measure.

Là l'esprit n'a de corps ni de couleurs non plus,
D'avoir lineamens moins encore au surplus,
D'avoir superficie on n'en voyt traict ny ligne,
Temongnage qu'il est de nature divine.
(*La Création, Chant quinzième*, 437)

Even though D'Aubigné's verses representing the soul and spirit suggest his desire to successfully represent them by means of pictorial images, they proved ultimately to be inadequate. The soul remained, with its spirit, a subject that could not be "reduyz au dedans d'une espace." Neither could the soul's site in the body be located although innumerable savants, himself included, had tried: ". . . beaucoup / De gens doctes se sont travaillez pour cognoystre / Où le siege d'icelle en ce corps pouroyt estre." Near the end of the last canto, D'Aubigné reflects on his attempt to describe the the soul's divine location and composition. He recognized that creating an image poetically required visual imagery, and that visual elements were as important to the poet as they were to the artist, but he realized that he would be unable fully to grasp the complexity of the body or understand the secret forces of the soul through poetry alone. True to his poetic art, he affirmed that the task was far too great to be accomplished within the confines of a sheet of paper. Furthermore, he knew that others would also fail trying to completely describe this *tableau*.

Quiquonques tascheroyt de vouloir achever
Ce qui est là compris & le tout observer
Il sembleroyt celuy qui veut en une page

Bien decrire un monde grand & large.
Je puys bien asseurer quant j'auroys entrepris
De rechercher le tout en ce tableau conpris
Pour en faire un rapport certain & bien fidelle
Mes ans seroyent trop cours pour entreprise telle.
(*La Création*, *Chant quinzième*, 442)

For D'Aubigné, painting, architecture and sculpture formed a bridge between the concrete and the abstract. Accordingly, they became a principal device for bringing his descriptions of the body and the soul into the proper light. The conscious visual quality of *La Création*, in which D'Aubigné depended heavily on portraits to describe the soul, resulted from the importance attributed both to visual art and to revealing man's anatomical structure during the Renaissance. His poem reflects the interdependence of verbal and visual art; his poetic language echoed the statement "ut pictura poesis." He consciously expressed himself in ways that surpassed the limits of language by inviting the reader to imagine and thereby to "see" a concrete visual experience.

2. Guillaume De Saluste Sieur Du Bartas, *Le Sixième jour*: Quattrocento triangle: *l'oeil*, *la main*, *le corps*

Du Bartas discusses both the visual nature of poetry and the role of the poet in a clear and circumspect manner in his *Brief Advertissement sur sa première et seconde Sepmaine* (1584).

> Davantage, puis qu'il est ainsi que la poésie est une parlante peinture, et que l'office d'un ingénieus escrivain est de marier le plaisir au proffit, qui trouvera estrange si j'ay rendu le païsage de ce tableau aussi divers que la nature mesme, . . .[62]

These remarks contain an interesting revelation in terms of Du Bartas' work and sixteenth-century poetry in general. They indicate that he consciously sought a visually eloquent poetic language in treating an exalted subject to move his readers. He conceived of poetry as being a *parlante peinture*, and saw himself as a poet rendering vivid portraitures in words. In describing what he considered to be the most important elements of his poetry, Du Bartas distinguished poetry from other forms of writing based on its pictorial charge; he deeply felt the influence of "Pictura on Poesis," and asserted that poetry was as much a picture of speech as a portrait might be of the body (hence the importance of harmony in both poetry and in God's living architectural construct, the human body). His remarks demonstrate his awareness of the intimate connections between the sister arts of poetry and art, and of the public acclaim for this affinity.[63] In this context, Du Bartas linked his interest in the relationship between his work and the visual arts with the exploration of the body through the three-level hierarchy of the "Quattrocento triangle": "l'oeil, la main et la chose à représenter (le monde, le corps). Cet objet que voit l'oeil, transcriptible par la main."[64]

Nowhere in Du Bartas' work is the concept of this hierarchy and the perception of poetry as *parlante peinture* more apparent than in his treatment of the creation of man's body in *Le Sixième jour* of the *Première Semaine*. This work consists of a poetic anatomy: a post-mortem (anatomical examination) in which painting and science interrelate with poetry to produce a poetic representation of man. Du Bartas believed that the poet's role was that of a prosector in the anatomy theater serving as a guide on a voyage of discovery into an unexplored land. He intended for his presentation to confirm the value of anatomical science and to demonstrate that prosection, integrated into a poetic structure, helped to display visually the body's natural world and to illuminate more accurately its secrets and the conspicuous power of God's infinite wisdom. Poised over the body, the poet asks dramatically: "Prendray-je la scalpelle . . . Pour voir . . . ?" The anonymous cadaver endures the poet-anatomist's scrutiny under the dissecting knife as Du Bartas declared.

> Hé! Quoy? N'est-il pas temps, n'est-il pas temps de voir
> Dans les secrets du corps le non-secret pouvoir
> D'un si parfait Ouvrier? Prendray-je la scalpelle
> Pour voir les cabinets de la double cervelle . . . ?
>
> (*Le Sixième jour*, vv. 641–44)

There is a persistent appeal to sight in Du Bartas' anatomy of the human body that is frequently stated in terms of established pictorial modes of beholding. In the following verses, in which he asserts that man is "Un tableau racourci, que . . . / Je veux ore tirer du pinceau de mes vers" (vv. 407–8), he attempts to convey the content of a picture by presenting the idea of his verses painting the body to demonstrate the exceptional descriptive power of his poetic art.

By mystically associating the words *pinceau*, *mains*, and *scalpelle*, and by the use of anatomical nomenclature such as *despecer*, *fendray*, and *despart*, Du Bartas suggests that the best way to comprehend the anatomy of man is through the artistry of the poet-anatomist-artist's "instruments à tous arts": the hands, which emulate God's by creating, and are thus capable of evoking His works, thus also making Du Bartas a *roi de la Création*.[65] He assumes the role of the Creator because this anatomy is conducted within the framework of the biblical Creation.

Mains, qui du corps humain tracez la pourtraiture,
Oublirez-vous les mains, chambrieres de nature,
Singes de l'Eternel, instruments à tous arts,
Et pour sauver nos corps non soudoyez soudars,
De nos conceptions diligentes greffieres,
Ministres de l'esprit, et du corps vivandieres?

(*Le Sixième jour*, vv. 623–28)

The poet becomes an inspired instrument of Creation, the *pinceau* or *scalpelle* that uses his eyes and hands as tools to examine and represent not only man's external features but also the micro aspects of this *petit monde*. Du Bartas conveyed a sense of control over the body by proposing that it be examined in this fashion. Yet in a manner similar to D'Aubigné's expression of an inability to portray the complexities of the body, Du Bartas feared that the body would defy representation, or that his mind would be unable to induce his hand to reproduce the body poetically. Displaying the secrets of its composition, he surmised, might require a more capable eye and a hand more *docte* than his *lourde-main* (v.479). Du Bartas implied that perhaps something more than artistry and anatomy were necessary to reveal poetic truth; he demonstrated considerable apprehension regarding such an anatomical undertaking.

Pourray-je desployer sur un docte fueillet
Ce Dedale subtil, cest admirable reth
Par les replis duquel l'esprit monte et devale,
Rendant sa faculté de vitale, Animale:

(*Le Sixième jour*, vv. 653–6)

Du Bartas surveyed and examined the body in just fifty-five verses of a 1055 line poem. He began with the three noble organs, and inspected related organs in descending order, i.e., *cervelle*, *coeur*, *poulmon*, *l'estomach*, and *foye*. Each is prefaced by a query such as *Prendray-je* (v. 643), *Pourray-je* (v. 653), *Descriray-je* (v. 660), *Fendray-je* (v. 669), and *Fendray-je* (v. 677). He finally abandons the endeavor, declaring

Mais non, je ne veux pas faire une ample reveue
Des membres que l'ouvrier desrobe à nostre veue.
Je ne veux despecer tout ce palais humain:
Car ce brave projet requiert la docte main
Des deux fils d'AEsculape, et le labouré style
Du disert Galien, ou du haut Herophile
Par cest eschantillon il me suffit d'avoir
Tellement quellement monstré le sainct pouvoir

(*Le Sixième jour*, vv. 699–706)

Even though he declined to anatomize the body thoroughly, Du Bartas imparted a sense of the mystery of the unopened body by forming an image of its inner reality that was concealed from the light of knowledge until the poet anatomist audaciously exposed it within the perspective of God's *non-secret pouvoir*.

Du Bartas drew poetry and painting even closer together when he tried to depict the creation of woman's body. He borrowed the technical language of the artist to provide an impressive example of the adage *ut pictura poesis* that transformed the reader into an observer who viewed woman through the medium of a written portrait.[66] Du Bartas distanced himself from contemporary medical practices by attempting to describe a beautiful woman admiringly without presenting individual details of her physical structure.

> Vous qui dans ce Tableau, parmi tant de pourtraits,
> Du Roy des animaux contemplez les beaux traits,
> Çà çà tournez un peu et vostre oeil et vostre ame,
> Et, ravis, contemplez les beaux traits de la femme,
>
> (*Le Sixième jour*, vv. 945–48)

As the representation of woman gains momentum in this passage, the reader-observer is distracted and discomfited by a vision of a surgeon removing diseased members of a male body. Du Bartas used distinct medical imagery to equate the *Tout-puissant* with the *Medecin*. This is later reinforced by a vision of a rib being removed from Adam's body to create woman. Du Bartas offers a double perspective of Adam as *l'amant* and Eve as *l'aimee*: "Qu'on ne peut discerner l'amant d'avec l'aimee" (v. 976).

> Comme le Medecin, qui desire trencher
> Quelque membre incurable, avant que d'aprocher
> Les glaives impiteux de la part offensee,
> Endort le patient d'une boisson glacee,
> Puis sans nulle douleur, guidé d'usage et d'art,
> Pour sauver l'homme entier, il en coupe une part:
> . . .
> Bref si bien engourdit et son corps et son ame
> Que sa chair sans douleur par ses flancs il entame
> Qu'il en tire une coste, et va d'elle formant
> La mere des humains, gravant si dextrement
> Tous les beaux traits d'Adam en la coste animee,
>
> (*Le Sixième jour*, vv. 961–66, 971–75)

Instead of describing the woman's physical composition, Du Bartas turns to a disappointing traditional presentation of a notion of beauty, one constituted simply of an enumeration of the body's parts and certain identifiable feminine characteristics.

> Bien vray toutesfois qu'elle a l'oeil plus riant,
> Le teint plus delicat, le front plus attrayant,
> Le menton net de poil, la parole moins forte,
> Et que deux monts d'yvoire en son sein elle porte.
> (*Le Sixième jour*, vv. 977–80)

We have seen how Du Bartas, inspired by the relationship between poetry and art, used pictorial terminology—his *parlante peinture*—to explore the anatomical structure of the male body and unveil the sensuality of the female body. However, his anatomical descriptions enabled the reader to identify more closely with the male's anatomy than to the female's. Du Bartas pursued this perspective perhaps because anatomies of the female were rare in Renaissance medicine, and also because he considered himself to be privileged observer of the body and the appropriate bearer of the male "look," with the male body being the proper object of his gaze.

3. Joseph Du Chesne, *L'Anatomie du Petit Monde*: Satirical anatomy, "tantost des pieds jusqu'à la teste."

Joseph Du Chesne also considered himself to be a privileged observer of the body, although he turned his attention to a more overtly moralizing presentation of it in verses deriding society's faults. In *L'Anatomie*, Du Chesne turned the established popular model of anatomical dissection to his own didactic needs. He departed from the objective and more anatomically correct (factual) views found particularly in D'Aubigné's work, and from the examination of the marvels of God's handiwork found in Creation narrative. In fact, Du Chesne only borrowed a skeleton framework from Creation. He attempted instead to convey a satirical and morally didactic message that focused clearly and graphically on the aftermath of the Fall. His interest in anatomizing the body was only partly medically motivated. He intended, rather, to present a serious religious and moral anatomy ("une petite Anatomie spirituelle de l'homme") which focused on mankind's corruption. Du Chesne proclaimed:

> . . . je declare l'usage depravé des parties de ceste creature la plus acomplie de toutes avant le peché, & maintenant la plus corrompue & miserable depuis sa rebellion (f. 2v).

He hoped that the poem would be taken seriously because the substance was Christian and therefore worthy of attention.

> L'argument donc de ceste matiere estant chrestien il sera treuvé bon comme je croi de toutes personnes qui ont quelque pieté, & crainte du Seigneur (f.2v).

In the *Odelette* (*épître*), which serves as preface to *L'Anatomie*, Du Chesne invited readers to examine the corrupted functions of the body.

Qui veut voir de chaque partie
Du corps l'office perverti,
Et comme l'homme est abruti,
Regarde mon Anatomie.

(*Odelette*, f. 3v)

The presentation of the body in the *Odelette* conforms loosely to the structure required in a conventional anatomy; its fourteen quatrains unite to form a rapid head-to-toe representation of the body (the *cerveau* with the five senses, the *coeur*, *poulmons* with the arteries and veins, the *entrailles*, and the *pieds & jambes*). The final verses introduce Du Chesne in his role as poet-prosector. The entry into the body is effected poetically, with the verses serving as the poet-prosector's precision instrument. Du Chesne's use of medical vocabulary demonstrates that he possessed a certain sophistication in handling surgical instruments.

VOILA, mon DE BROSSES, en somme
Ce que tantost vous fera voir
De mes vers l'afilé rasoir
Incisant les membres de l'homme

(f. 4v.)[67]

The *Odelette* also reflects Du Chesne's preoccupation with themes that appear throughout *L'Anatomie*. He subjects his audience to solemn warnings by dwelling obsessively on the corrupted functions of the body, its vices, follies and manifestations of physical impurity.

Although the sections of *L'Anatomie* that treat actual anatomical inquiries are brief (and interspersed with reprobation), they nonetheless elucidate Renaissance anatomical procedures. They set a clear goal for the anatomy lesson that differs little from present day post-mortem examinations: the discovery of remedies by determining the causes of disease and death. The surgeon explains the purpose of the anatomy in the *huitain* below. The inquiry occurs within defined limits determined by the notion of a fixed relationship between man and God. Du Chesne was obviously enthusiastic about acquiring anatomical knowledge. It is a lesson in which he seeks remedies for the living.

Des morts on fait l'anatomie
Pour les maux conoistre au dedans
Ausquels sont sujets les vivans
Afin que lon y remedie:
O mon Dieu fai moi donc la grace
Qu'incise l'homme en la façon
Que t'y aprene la leçon

Que tu permets que je lui face.

(*L'Anatomie*, *Huitain*, VIII, f. 6v)

However, much of the interest in *L'Anatomie* lies in the way in which the poet depicts a different aspect of the anatomical picture. His main theme is the inevitable death and putrefaction of the human body. Secondarily, *L'Anatomie* is an anti-Catholic tirade and a polemic against the dissension in France caused by the religious wars. More broadly, his invective is a much wider attack against mankind's injustices, immoralities and frivolities.

Oyez donques mes chants vous Princes de ce monde
Qui estes demi dieux & en terre, & en l'onde,
Vous qui faites trembler par vos foudres hideux
Razans quelque cité, l'air, la terre & les cieux,
. . .
Vous qui robe-portez, toi peuple, & vous en somme
Hommes mortels qui tous estes or' assemblez
Pour avec le rasoir de mes vers afilez
Les membres plus pourris voir decouper de l'homme:
Quand vous verrez tantost des pieds jusqu'à la teste
Tant de vices en l'homme & de corruption,
En vous mesme jugeans qu'il n'y a rien de bon
Au moins qu'à l'avenir d'y pourvoir on s'apreste.

(*L'Anatomie*, *Huitains*, III, V, VII) (f. 5v 6r)

Du Chesne declared satirically that instead of producing a series of physiological observations traditionally ordered (*a capite ad calcem*), that he would reverse the order and seek a different knowledge about man's fabric, one "tantost des pieds jusqu'à la teste." In reality, he followed the classical order by beginning with the *cerveau*, providing an anatomically correct description of it as "un moiste cerveau / Entouré de deux peaux & d'une osseuse boëste," and examining its fragility and the consequent vulnerability of man's body.

O fragile l'estui qui telle chose enserre!
Homme, juge en cela ta grande infirmité
Car ce rare thresor, las te peut estre osté
Pour un vent par un rien qui tout à coup t'aterre

(*L'Anatomie*, *Huitain*, IX, f. 6v)

Each organ (*membre*) and its use are examined in the ensuing verses. The *coeur*, ". . . la fournaise / De toute afection mauvaise"; the *poulmons*, "Pour chanter des choses profanes"; followed by the *foye*, which he stops to admire, taking the opportunity to reaffirm his status as prosector.

Prendrai-je le rasoir pour decouper de rang
Le foye chaleureux l'origine des veines,
Qui, comme des ruisseaux decoulans des fonteines,
S'espanchent par le corps pour l'abruver de sang?
De ce membre aumosnier admirons la nature,

(*L'Anatomie*, *Huitain*, XXIII, f. 9v)

Du Chesne achieved an effect of revulsion against the human body in dissecting the spleen (*ratelle*), by employing a battery of words that describe the decay and stench to which the human frame is susceptible.

Ca de mon pointu scarpelle
Homme, j'incise ta ratelle:
He Dieu quelle vilaine lie
Contraire à l'Eternelle vie
De peché toute infecte en sort,
Plus puamment puante & noire
Que celle que la mort fait boire
Aux mortels, du stix sur le bord.

(*L'Anatomie*, *Huitain* XXVI, f. 10r)

The poet's tactile experience of the intestines (*boyaux*), further expands this olfactory vocabulary and makes it clear that he, was more than simply an observer of the body. Du Chesne had first hand knowledge of post-mortems, unlike D'Aubigné and Du Bartas. His use of "j'incise" demonstrates a dissection in progress, not merely insinuated as in Du Bartas' "Prendray-je."

Ou toucher aux puans boyaux
Qui ressemblent à serpenteaux,
Quelle est la main, empunaisie
Qui ne fust de leur vilenie?

(*L'Anatomie*, *Huitain* XXVIII, f. 10v)

Overall, Du Chesne propounded a rather distinctive view of the role of sense perception and anatomy in relation to the knowledge of bodily functions. Medical representations of the five senses offered Du Chesne ample opportunity to inlay religious conceptions and promote the Christian ideal of mastering communications between the exterior and interior of the body via these *portes*. It is rather interesting to read Du Chesne's satirical description of the senses which offers a far more interesting social depiction of sixteenth century anatomy than that portrayed by the other poets studied here.

Among the orifrices to be closely watched, according to Du Chesne, is the mouth (*bouche*), which in conjunction with the tongue, is seen as a site of sinful gluttony and loquacity. Both may be linked to Du Chesne's use of the theme of the aftermath of the Fall.

L'homme gourmand à toute heure s'adonne
Faisant son Dieu de sa bouche gloutonne.
. . .
La langue qui va blasphemant,
La langue, qui mesdit, qui ment,
Depuis qu'on lui lasche le frain
Est la perte du genre humain,

(*L'Anatomie*, *Huitains*, XXXVII, XLII) (f. 12r 13r)

To control the orifrices of the body, Du Chesne recommended a religious prescription rather than a medical one (prescribing, for example, service to God and reading the Bible). Yet, he proceeded to echo sixteenth century medical concerns while giving moral and religious prescriptions for the body. Du Chesne noted that imprudent ingestion of alimentary substances (gluttony) could damage and weaken the body. He recommended prudent ingestion and a regulated diet. In fact, dietary regulation was considered one of a physician's duties and was included in medical textbooks from the fourteenth through the early sixteenth centuries.[68]

L'homme, entre tous les animaux,
Est plus sujet à divers maux,
Pour la diversité des mets
Que dedans son friand palez
Le glouton engoufre à toute heure,
Sans tenir reigle ne mesure:

(*L'Anatomie*, *Huitain*, XXXVIII, f. 12v)

In each of the *huitains* devoted to individual sense perceptions, Du Chesne applied the same technique and employed little plastic description of the anatomy. The *huitains* serve more generally as an attack on the general social and moral shortcomings of mankind which Du Chesne considered to be most important. His castigation involves much anti-courtier invective, especially against luxuries (see below under Gender for anti-courtisane censure). The concluding *huitains* recall Medieval medical themes, especially that of Alain de Lille, in which the body is reduced by *la mort farouche*, its members ultimately devoured by worms.[69]

Ou sont ces tendons roïdes forts
Et ces muscles qui tout le corps
Te composoyent d'une figure
La plus admirable en nature?
Ou sont ces nerfs qui sentiment
Te donnoyent & tout mouvement,
Et tant d'autres vaisseaux divers?
Ils sont dans le ventre des vers.

(*L'Anatomie*, *Huitain* XLVIII, f. 14v)

In content, Du Chesne's *L'Anatomie* is very different from the other poetic anatomies examined in this section. He has no intention to be unbiased or objective in describing and analyzing the various parts of the human body; his purpose is admonish. He is deeply interested in spouting anti-Catholic, anti-mondain, and anti-courtly invective. He is detached from any vision of wholeness or harmony of the body as found in Du Bartas or D'Aubigné; his learned gaze concentrates rather on fragmented phenomena of the body. Du Chesne's poetic ''je,'' found in his ''j'incise,'' contributes significantly to the impression of lived experience. The *persona* Du Chesne creates represents an individualized speaker immersed in the sordid realities of the body. By means of this poetic voice Du Chesne not only incorporated the world of the Renaissance physician prosecting the body into his poem, but introduced social and courtly experience as well.

In form, Du Chesne's work recalls the legacy of poets such as Villon and Clément Marot, primarily in his use of eight-line stanzas or *huitains*.[70] Several of his themes (e.g., dwelling on the death and putrefaction of the body) are representative of poets writing in the first half of the sixteenth century. However, I do not regard *L'Anatomie* as being an eccentric interpretation of the sixteenth century anatomy, but rather as a variation of a conscious effort to produce scientific poetry that observed man and focused on his social identity, particularly on the manifestations of the vices of immorality and luxury.

The next section is devoted to the questions of biological sexuality and social identities, and concentrates on further manifestations of human weakness through an analysis of the Creation poets' representations of men's and women's bodies.

Gender: The Sexually Differentiated Body

> Le sexe n'est autre chose que la difference du masle et de la femelle: en laquelle faut considerer que la femme a tousjours moins de chaleur que l'homme, aussi qu'elle a quelques parties peu differentes, et situées en autre lieu que l'homme . . .
>
> (Paré, *Oeuvres* ''Introduction à la chirurgie'' Chapitre XI, 60)

Many Creation poets were compelled to differentiate by gender in their work because Genesis, which served as their model, describes the whole world as being gendered (''male and female created he them'' [1.27]).[71] Aristotle and Galen were the most important authorities on the physiological distinction between male and female, yet no privileged discourse offered a definitive method to distinguish them.[72] Their ideas were reinforced by a number of Renaissance physicians who, like Paré, perpetuated the belief that woman "a tousjours moins de chaleur que l'homme," and that she had "quelques parties peu differentes, et situées en autre lieu que l'homme."

Creation poems provided models of traditional texts produced by the male-authored poetic system in sixteenth century Europe. As such, they contain the male conception of the inequality of the sexes. Three poets, Du Bartas, D'Aubigné and Du Chesne, anatomized the body in their Creation poems. Each subjected the body of the male to varying degrees of sexual examination, and all except D'Aubigné (in *La Sorcière*) avoided examining woman anatomically.[73] Although female anatomy is largely excluded from their consideration, it appears obliquely through notions of a fixed sexual identity. Each poet suggests in different ways that the female body, and thus the feminine identity, was more a construct imposed by social organization.

D'Aubigné, who interprets gender in *La Création* largely as a matter of dissimilar genitalia, provides a clear example of gender assymetry exhibited in Creation poetry. His anatomical investigation involves a body that he gradually endows with a gendered (male) identity. In so doing, he provides an excellent example of the emergence of gender-based roles derived from Aristotle's binarism.[74] The anatomical presentation in *La Création* begins with descriptions of three noble organs of life: "Troys choses sont au corps dont le reste despend, / . . . le foye . . . / le coeur & le cerveau." D'Aubigné then introduces a fourth, the testes, which identify the body as a male.

On en peut dire quatre à bon droyt, car du corps
Ce n'est rien ou bien peu, les testiculles hors:
Non qu'en particullier sans eux n'ayt habitude,
Mays bien pour conserver l'espace & multitude.
D'autre part on les tient plus nobles que le coeur,
Quoy qu'il soyt le motif & don de la vigueur,
A cause qu'ils font l'home acord, promp & à destre,
Et le coeur simplement luy donne vie & estre
Retranchez de ce corps, quoy qu'il soyt masle né,
Cela le rend confus, couhard, effeminé,
Sans barbe, sans couleur, sans voix digne d'un homme,
Comme l'effect monstre en cil qu'ennucque on nomme.

(*La Création*, *Chant Unzieme*, 406)

The poem defines male identity in terms of virility, and denotes a number of gender characteristics associated with maleness, including the active role in generation. At the same time, D'Aubigné revealed that the male state, supposedly made secure by the laws of Nature's hierarchy, was precariously balanced, contingent on the testes, and could verge on becoming "womanish." Maleness signified virility and the exclusion of all traces of disorder or unmanliness from the body. Removal of the testes meant destruction of the robust and masculine constitution, and rendered the male body *confus*, *couhard*, or *effeminé*.

D'Aubigné infers that females are inferior and hierarchically subordinate to males. He ascribes numerous negative qualities to females, and remarks that they lack specific attributes, notably the male's fourth noble organ. He also implies that they lack *couleur* and are thus *confus* and *couhard*. The poet does extol women's scriptural virtues, but he reinforces their negative attributes by his terminology, suggesting that females are incapable of rational choice or fixity of purpose. The "scientific" foundation for these assertions was the belief that woman was man without *ratio*, a castration allegory that identifies the phallus with reason.

D'Aubigné deals with Adam's creation in the *Chant Unzieme* of *La Création*, subtitled "De la Creation de l'home et dignité d'iceluy," but ignores Eve's. However, the female body appears obliquely in the *Chant* in a discussion of the *souverain droyt* of God to bestow names on all creatures, and man's right to name his spouse (in nuptial ceremonies), his offspring (at birth), and others in similar situations of subordination. D'Aubigné weaves a poetic image from these examples in which he reinforces woman's social status and corporeal subjugation to man, and implies control over all conquered bodies, just as the the warrior claims the vanquished body of his opponent. By naming his wife, the man thereby gives her his identity, and also the physical *marques* of the conqueror (e.g., *le nom & la loy*).

Affin de l'introduyre & mieux le maintenir
    En ce souverain droyt, faison ores venir
    Tous animaux vers luy & que tous il les nomme,
    En signe qu'ilz sont tous asubjectiz à l'homme.
Ainsi comme le pere a ceste autorité
    De nommer son enfant à sa nativité,
    Ou quand par mariage une femme se lie
    Prend du mary le nom & le sien elle oublie,
Ou bien comme un guerrier, soyt Grand, Seigneur & Roy,
    Vainceur donne au vaincu & le nom & la loy,
    Tout ainsi qu'il luy plaist, toutes marques en somme
    D'une subjection dessus tous ceux qu'on nomme:

(*La Création*, *Chant Unzieme*, 403–04)

As mentioned above, D'Aubigné does anatomize the female body in *La Sorcière*, a poem only indirectly related to his Creation poetry, focusing on images of female sexuality and prostitution. He represents the "grotesque" body of a witch. The organs of her aberrant anatomy lack the composition and proportions of a normal healthy body. He confirms this by discovering by means of tactile experience that she lacks the three noble organs.

Cherchons où est le foie . . . en autre endroit . . . point, point,
Vous luy cherchez du noble, elle n'en avait point.
Au moins où est son coeur? mais quant à la main j'y passe
Je ne rencontre rien que du fiel en sa place.
Ouvrons luy le cerveau: voicy d'autres poisons,
Il souffre cacochisme & est plain de poisons.

(*La Sorcière*, vv. 73–78)

In contraposition to Paré's statement that "la femme a tousjours moins de chaleur que l'homme," D'Aubigné endows her with a body so *chalereuse*, resulting from her hot choleric temperament, that several organs are charred: "Ses rognons sont brulez, . . . / Et son sang monstre bien qu'elle fut chaleureuse" (vv.79–80). Furthermore, he suggests that her extreme constitution is poisonous, and that the bad humors in her own body have poisoned her.[75]

An essential aspect of D'Aubigné's anatomical examination of the witch is his representation of her sexual body. He endows her with a *matrice* that confirms her sex and which, upon dissection, discloses a twin pregnancy.

Ouvrez luy la matrice: O! elle avoit dedans
Deux germes commancez de deux pauvres enfans!

(*La Sorcière*, vv. 81–82)

Renaissance medicine related the occurence of multiple births to an abnormal proportion of the semen (*superabondance de matiere*).[76] This image of multiple embryos may also be linked to certain connections between female sexuality and witchcraft, and to insatiable carnal lusts to which witches were presumed to be subject.[77] Several components of female sexual deviance are noted in *La Sorcière* even before the anatomical examination begins. D'Aubigné confirmed the sexual identity of this witch *qua* prostitute, and provided her with a long history of perversion and lust by the use of terms such as *la sorcière*, *putain*, and *maquerelle*: "Putain dés le berceau, dés saize ans maquerelle".

D'Aubigné resolved the dilemma of female degeneracy and disease represented in the witch's body by terminating the encounter through a denial of her female sexual body. He leaves her corpse to putrify as a symbol of disorder and disintegration in society.

Mes amis, je m'en fuis, car je meurs sans mourir.[78]
Laissons ce cors aux champs des orages pourrir,
Il troublera tout l'aer d'odeur & de desordre.

(*La Sorcière*, vv. 85–87)

In contrast to D'Aubigné's *La Sorcière*, Joseph Du Chesne did not directly treat distinctively female anatomy in his *L'Anatomie*. Sexuality, however, and specifically prostitution, appear in accompanying sonnets. Woman appears in *La Prodigalité*, where she is defined largely by her social relationship to males, because Du Chesne wishes to comment upon the loose morals that seem to have existed especially at court. Noble and ignoble women alike are represented fleetingly as the "courtisane au lict," *la garce*, and symbolized by the *bordeau*. These female figures are used as examples to caution against vanity, immorality and extravagance (Fig. 1.4., An old man embracing a nude courtesan, with a fool and death watching the scene).

Les vestemens, le jeu, le bourdeau, & la pance,
Le drap d'or, le velours, les cartes & les detz,
La courtisane au lict, en table force metz,
. . .

Le marchant, le gaignant, la garce & provoyeur,
. . .
O prodigues enfans ne suyvez donc mon train:
Qui m'a tout despouillé, qui m'a mis à la faim?
Les vestemens, le jeu, le bordeau & la pance.

(*La Prodigalité*, vv. 1–3, 9, 12–14)

In Du Chesne's examination of the sexuality and pathological anatomy of the male in *L'Anatomie*, the prosected male body represents society in its most debased and diseased condition. He allows a significant image of society to emerge by illustrating the oppositions noble-ignoble. To Du Chesne, the greatest single source of mankind's depraved condition and adversity was what Renaissance medicine and most of his peers considered to be the fourth noble organ.

L'homme, l'artere aorte & les deux parastates,
Les reins & les vailleaux expellens, preparans,
Le dartos, l'erythree & les retors Prostates,
Sont de tes gransmalheurs les beaus premiers parens:
Il eust bien mieux valu, semence viperine,
Que tu n'eusse onc veu du beau jour la clarté,
Qu'ores par la laideur de ton iniquité,
En eternelle nuict finir ton origine.[79]

(*L'Anatomie*, *Huitain*, XXIX, f. 10v)

Du Chesne employed imagery of generation to present his reactions to the atrocities perpetrated in the civil wars and to dispense moral guidance in *L'Anatomie*. He noted that amid plants and animals generating their kind in the natural world ("Car toute chose qui vit / L'une espece l'autre

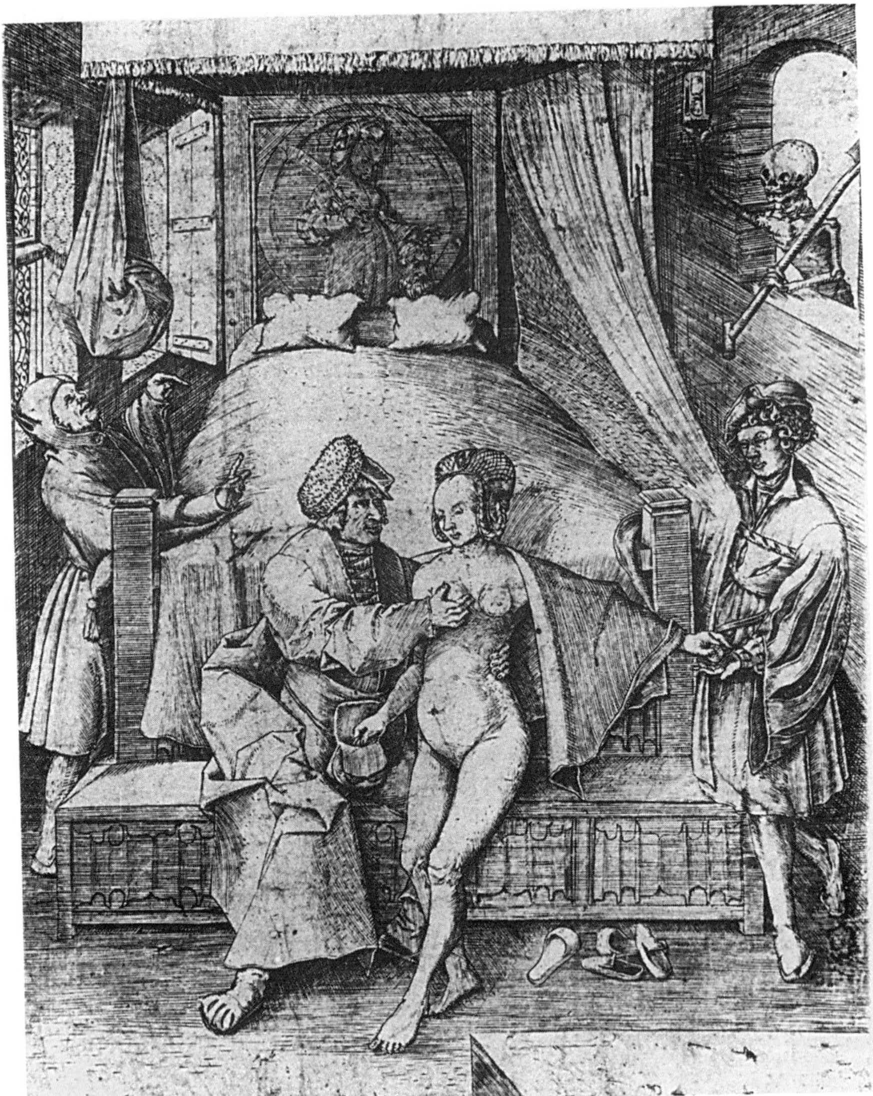

Figure 1.4 Engraving of *An old man embracing a nude courtesan.* After Lucas van Leyden, 16th century. (Photo: The Warburg Institute, London.)

produit.''), the *flancs* of man produced only aberrant offspring intent upon destroying each other.

Mais les flancs de l'homme, entre tous
Les animaux, ores produisent
Au lieu d'hommes des loups garous
Tous nouveaux, qui s'entredestruisent.

(*L'Anatomie*, *Huitain*, XXX, f. 11r)[80]

Du Chesne did not focus on biological sexuality to seek the truth of the body's physical condition. Instead, he used the polarity between normality and abnormality to illustrate contemporary social and cultural circumstances which he condemned.

In contrast to Du Chesne's discernible plan of social identity, Du Bartas had quite a different view of male and female sexual identity in *Le Sixième jour*. He focused on the normal male anatomy. He presented it in a somewhat idealized manner, employing the image of a labyrinth to compare the seminal vesicles to the *replis* found in the brain.[81]

Pourray-je desployer sur un docte fueillet
Ce Dedale subtil, cest admirable reth
. . .
Tout ainsi que le sang et les esprits errans
Par le chemin courbé des vaisseaux preparans
D'un cours entortillé s'elabourent, se cuisent
Et en sperme fecond peu à peu se reduisent?

(*Le Sixième jour*, vv. 654–55, 657–60)

However, no clear image of the female anatomy emerges from Du Bartas' representation of the woman. Her appearance is so idealized that her physical and anatomical presence virtually disappears. As noted, it is found only in expressions such as those denoting her *rares beautez* (v. 986), and in those that fleetingly describe a universal physical appearance.

Predictably, there is gender asymetry in Creation poems because they conform to a generalized patriarchal model. However, even though the poets examined in this section were unwilling, perhaps unconfortable, about examining the biological body of woman, they did examine the male body in concise ways. Overall, they offer valuable ways to study certain medical practices and systems of social relations in sixteenth-century France.

Creation poets enlightened their readers about the body's poetic truth: the unknown, the ineffable, and the divine mysteries and secrets of its universe. They acknowledged that their treatment of the human body was a privileged one in which they viewed themselves symbolically as the King of Creation because they knew the secrets of nature (or at least how to set about discovering them) and thus could create a man. They considered the body, which was an embodied object over which the poet had control, to be the point of departure for reflecting on man's nature; its composition was viewed as being inherently pictorial; vision provided the basic metaphor for interpreting it as a class of portraits. The body's secrets could be revealed by opening it with surgical instruments and reading it by means of visual terminology. Thus he could observe, contemplate and experience the intimate interior as well as the exposed exterior. Yet poets discovered vast complexity in their seemingly simple representation of the body's physical inner secrets. They often encountered their own inability or reluctance to express it adequately in words, fearing they would be unable to represent the body's intricacies satisfactorily.

However, as we have seen in this survey, anatomy alone failed to satisfy the scrupulous poet desirous of fashioning anatomically idealized copies. He searches further for his representations, beyond the visible and material nature of the body into the idealized forms of poetic creativity, and focuses on the social identity of his subjects for more clarity.

Chapter II
Health and Disease:
Joachim du Bellay's *Les Regrets*[82]

When Joachim Du Bellay went to Rome in 1553 as an intendant in the service of the French crown in Cardinal Jean du Bellay's retinue, he believed that he was entering a career that would bring him fame and fortune. But he was quickly disillusioned. He became an unhappy exile from his beloved France, for which he suffered a profound nostalgia. The following verses record his aspirations on leaving for Italy and his subsequent disenchantment.

Je me feray sçavant en la philosophie,
    En la mathematique, & medicine aussi,
    Je me feray legiste, & d'un plus hault souci
    Apprendray les secrets de la theologie:
Du luth & du pinceau j'ebateray ma vie,
    De l'escrime & du bal. Je discourois ainsi,
    Et me vantois en moy d'apprendre tout cecy,
    Quand je changeay la France au sejour d'Italie.
O beaux discours humains! je suis venu si loing,
    Pour m'enrichir d'ennuy, de vieillesse, & de soing,

(*Les Regrets*, S. 32, vv. 1–10)

Du Bellay referred to his various artistic, political, scientific, philosophical and medical ambitions in the *Regrets*, but he was especially attracted by medicine and philosophical traditions, which consequently played important roles in the composition of many sonnets. Lexical evidence in the sonnet sequence reveals that he was interested in schooling himself in medical knowledge, i.e., the study of humoral psychology, which includes astrological conventions, the four primary humoral types, their corresponding planetary dominations, and their relationships to the body.[83] A noteworthy example of the poet's medical interests is found in references in sonnet 74 to his awareness of his own complexional nature (''Aussi ma qualité ne baisse ny ne monte / Car je ne suis subject qu'à ma complexion [vv. 7–8]), and in the fact that he learned to "Cognoistre les humeurs" (S. 85, v. 9) in Rome.[84]

In another sonnet, which relates to sixteenth-century scientific and medical theories, and in which he exhibits considerable interest in planetary influences, the poetic *persona* interprets experiences that occurred prior to his departure for Italy.[85] Du Bellay considered the year, the month, the day, the hour and the instant all to be unpropitious when he set out for Italy ("malheureux l'an, le mois, le jour, l'heure, & le poinct" [S. 25 v. 1]). He identified malevolent celestial influences when Mars and Saturn were in conjunction that portended evil events on his departure. They crystallized when he sprained his ankle "sur le sueil de l'huis, . . . / Je me blessay le pied sortant de ma maison" (S. 25, vv. 13–14).[86]

Vrayment d'un bon oiseau guidé je ne fus point,
   Et mon coeur me donnoit assez signifiance
   Que le ciel estoit plein de mauvaise influence,
   Et que Mars estoit lors à Saturne conjoint.
Cent fois le bon advis lors m'en voulut distraire,
   Mais tousjours le destin me tiroit au contraire:

(*Les Regrets*, S. 25, vv. 5–10)

Medicine and humoral psychology are both found in one of the most prominent themes woven into this sonnet sequence: a finely constructed perception of a "morose, ill, homesick, and self-pitying" poetic *persona*.[87] Du Bellay promoted contemplation through melancholy to examine the textual body of this *persona*, to record changes in its physiology, to express his feelings about Italy, and to assess people in general. The physiological assumptions that he used to produce this *persona* include the concept of the Renaissance melancholic disposition, derived in part from Petrarchan traditions, by means of which he "veut surtout convaincre le lecteur de son malheur." Furthermore, melancholia, whether or not influenced by Petrarch, provided the superstructure for the textual body of the poetic *persona* in the *Regrets*. The melancholic physiology and psychology are both inscribed in the sonnets through identifiable "portraits" that the poet developed by exploiting the structures of illness and infirmity. The symptoms that Du Bellay ascribes to the textual body are medically established and philosophically identifiable features of melancholy, a disease that had its origins in Greek medicine.[89]

Melancholy, which also frequently denoted illnesses that involved all four humors, was an all-encompassing term for illness in the Renaissance. Du Bellay considered it to be both a psychological condition and a physical disorder, and used it to reveal an ill-disposed, unbalanced, aging and debilitated body.[90] He presented various contemporary medical views on the disease as well as the ecclesiastical interpretation, in which it was viewed as a vice.

Du Bellay also accepted, as did other Pléiade poets, Florentine philosopher Marsilio Ficino's belief that the "melancholy of great men was simply a metonomy for Plato's divine *mania*."[91] This alternative conception of melancholy as a divine gift that enhanced the creative capacity of the artist and writer came to be considered a fundamental prerequisite for genius possessed by many men of letters. Du Bellay found this theory of artistic creation useful in highlighting and valorizing the body.

Satire and melancholy exhibit an affinity in Du Bellay's sonnet sequence because he used them as frameworks for observing and evaluating human behavior. Both enabled the poet to express himself about matters that concerned him directly, and provided an effective way to depict the body textually. Du Bellay gained remarkable latitude in the *Regrets* by understanding and deploying the signifying systems of the realms of satire, which he directed at the Romans and the Papal court, and the elegiac, which he used to convey his ennuis and melancholy. Interestingly, L. Wierenga suggests that the same inspiration led to both.

> Du point du vue de la poétique humaniste, il est anachronique de parler d'une inspiration élégiaque qui s'ajouterait à l'inspiration satirique: la satire, en tant que genre, comporte l'observation, la passion, la mélancolie, l'ironie, la plainte.[92]

Furthermore, the melancholic was always thought to project his feelings outwardly more radically than other humoral types. And because of the black bile connected with the humoral disposition he was equally inclined to see evil in what he believed to be a vice-ridden world. Du Bellay articulated the portrait of the poetic *persona* as well as his satire of the Romans and the Papal court at least partly through the poetic theme of melancholia. He used satire sharply, eloquently and effectively to express his complaints and to console himself in his exile.[93]

> De quelque mal un chacun se lamente,
> mais les moiens de plaindre sont divers:
> J'ay, quant à moy, choisi celuy des vers
> Pour desaigrir l'ennuy qui me tormente.
> C'est pourquoy d'une douce satyre
> Entremeslant les espines aux fleurs,
> Pour ne fascher le monde de mes pleurs,
> J'appreste icy le plus souvent à rire.
>
> (*A Monsieur D'Avanson*, vv. 77–84)

Melancholy, or more accurately the theme of illness found in the lexicon of the elegiac pieces of the *Regrets*, aided Du Bellay in his satirical orientation. Although the term melancholia never appears in the sonnet sequence (He classified this illness under the rubric *ceste maladie* [S. 59 v. 5]), the melancholic disposition and conspicuous symptoms of a chronic non-febrile disorder are portrayed throughout. The poet also connected the textual body's physical and mental states with the world as he interpreted it.[94]

I examine in the following pages Du Bellay's sophisticated treatment of what Gilbert Gadoffre calls a ''mélancolie stylisée,'' which is expressed in the *Regrets* both as a physical reality and as a form of mental disorder.[95] The discourse of melancholia validates the textual body and becomes a culturally acceptable and legitimate representation of the identity of that poetic body while also allowing Du Bellay to discuss the torment of his exile.

To facilitate the examination of this ostensibly stylized melancholia, I have divided the following section into a series of ''portraits'' of various types of ailments, most of which appear in the first 130 sonnets.[96] They serve to characterize the textual body and help to examine the ''melancholy of an exile . . . longing for his home in Anjou.''[97] I examine the textual body in these sonnets generally under the category of malady and melancholy, and then as represented by the following portraits: the signs of melancholy in the body (old age and youth), the disempowerment of ennui and idleness (activity and lethargy), the would-be scholar authority and subservience), and the mad poet creativity and stagnation). These sonnets also deal with the Papal court and the streets of Rome, and contain mockery and satiric complaints and compliments. However, I have limited my inquiry to specific representations of the poet's textual body, and to the symptomatology of melancholy when they relate to the creation or legitimation of that poetic *persona*.

The Textual Body: Malady and Melancholy

Among the corporeal discourses in the *Regrets*, Du Bellay uses the theme of health and illness as a creative stratagem and as a stimulating way to examine the body of the poet's *persona*. As Terence Cave observes in reference to Rabelais' works, but which applies equally well to the model of the body constructed in the *Regrets*,

> Many tricks can be played with this model of the body; all of them have to do with the fabrication of a grounding or a set of oppositions health-disease, inner-outer) by means of which discourse can claim authenticity.[98]

A striking example of this "inner-outer" opposition is found in the beautifully expressed lamentation of sonnet 52, in which the body becomes a paradigm for physiological unity and functioning. Du Bellay established in this sonnet his acquaintance with the current physiological theory that melancholy was purged as tears through the eyes. "Si les larmes servoient de remede au malheur, / Et le pleurer pouvoit la tristesse arrester" (S. 52, vv. 1–2).[99] He also relates the theory that the heart manufactured tears that reached the brain by a circuitous route before falling upon the chest, where they evaporate or are reabsorbed by the body.[100]

> Le coeur fait au cerveau ceste humeur exhaler,
> Et le cerveau la fait par les yeux devaller,
> Mais le mal par les yeux ne s'allambique pas.
> Dequoy donques nous sert ce fascheux larmoyer?
> De jetter comme on dit l'huile sur le foyer,
> Et perdre sans profit le repoz & repas.
>
> (*Les Regrets*, S. 52, vv. 9–14)

Du Bellay used the model of the body to exploit various roles played by the *persona*. They may be conveniently studied by examining polarities such as activity-lethargy, creative energy-stagnation, old age-youth, and authority-subservience. The traditions of melancholy provided the poet with a series of recognizable physiological portraits and psychological characterizations that enhanced these oppositions because the disease conformed readily to various definitions, as will be seen in the portraits that follow.

Signs of Melancholy in the Body: Old Age and Youth

Du Bellay viewed the body as an object with specific physiological characteristics, and thus subject to natural processes of aging and decay. However, he gave the body of the *persona* considerable symbolic significance in the *Regrets*. He also denoted its physical, mental and personality changes, and interpreted various physical symptoms that he associated with pain and, in particular, with his reaction to being in exile. A number of these symptoms may be related to melancholy in the body, and were described by Robert Burton in *The Anatomy of Melancholy* (1621). Burton derived them from a variety of Classical and contemporary sources, as noted in the following passage. These symptoms, he wrote,

> are either universal or particular, . . . But to confine them, these general symptoms may be reduced to those of the body or the mind. Those usual signs appearing in the bodies of such as are melancholy be these, cold and dry, or they are hot and dry, as the humour is more or less adjust. . . . Hippocrates

in his book *de insania et melan.* reckons up these signs, that they are "lean, withered, hollow-eyed, look old, wrinkled, harsh, much troubled with . . . little or no sleep, and that interrupt, terrible and fearful dreams."[101]

Moreover, because autumn is the season "in which risith the black colre," it is also when men who are passing from their prime into the cold, dry autumn of their lives are particularly susceptible to melancholy.[102] In sonnet 21, Du Bellay refers to coldness and his "stile aussi lent, que lente est ma froideur" (S. 21 v. 8), thus inferring that his complexional nature was cold. Du Bellay's *persona* fits satisfactorily into the mold of the melancholic type considering the extent of his preoccupation with coldness, dryness, and winter, the auspices of the melancholy planet Saturn, which is by nature cold and dry, the house of Capricorn, which rules over melancholy, and, in general, his obsession with the passing of youth and the onset of aging to be found in the *Regrets*.

There are memorable references in the first 50 sonnets to old age and excessive self-pity in the poetic *persona*'s body. These are especially apparent in sonnets 35, 37, and 42, where they are associated with the theme of exile. Thus, sonnets that focus on aging also imply the body of the *persona*, who declares: "Je vieillis peu à peu sur l'onde Ausonienne" (S. 35 v. 12). His bitter exile has consumed the best years of his life. "Je veille ma franchise en prison se changer, / Et la fleur de mes ans en l'hyver de ma vie" (S. 37 vv. 13–14). He admits sadly that he has foolishly let his youth fade away. "Et que ce que j'estois plus estre je ne puis, / Aiant perdu mon temps, & ma jeunesse encore" (S. 42 v. 3–4). These examples indicate that Du Bellay created a *persona* preoccupied with age, for whom youth possessed an exaggerated significance. He created a personality prone to excessive sadness who is categorized as a melancholic by virtue of this characteristic.

Sonnet 28 also reveals various age-related physical symptoms of melancholy. The sonnet expresses Du Bellay's desire to record changes in the personality and physical constitution of the poetic *persona*. He recalls his farewell to a friend (Lahaye) before leaving France, and advice that he received to be the same on his return as when he left. His concept of his pre-departure *persona* did not change, but his body developed signs of afflictions, particularly aging. Although these characteristics are common in old age, they were also interpreted as being indications of melancholy, particularly in apparently premature aging.

Et tel comme je vins, je m'en retourne aussi:
Hors mis un repentir qui le coeur me devore,
Qui me ride le front, qui mon chef decolore,
Et qui me fait plus bas enfoncer le sourcy.

Ce triste repentir qui me ronge, & me lime,
Ne vient (car j'en suis net) pour sentir quelque crime
Mais pour m'estre trois ans à ce bord arresté:
(*Les Regrets*, S. 28, vv. 5–11)

Du Bellay interprets this corporeal unhealthiness as something that may be easily recognized outwardly, e. g., a scowl, a wrinkled brow and grey hair, but which also devours the internal organs. He attributed these undeserved afflictions not to any immoral conduct but to three years of abuse and poverty in Rome, which he blames for changing the outward appearance of the body to one appearing old, wrinkled and harsh. He also suggests sarcastically that Rome caused him to lose his hair.[103]

Heureux qui peult sans mal vivre l'aage d'un homme!
Heureux qui sans soucy peult garder son tresor!
Sa femme sans souspçon, & plus heureux encor'
Qui a peu sans peler vivre trois ans à Rome!
(*Les Regrets*, S. 94, vv. 11–14)

In another sonnet, however, in which Du Bellay incorporates humoral theory to characterize the body of the poet's *persona*, he claims that its fundamental nature did not change because its condition was based upon its temperament or natural complexion. ''Aussi ma qualité ne baisse ny ne monte, / Car je ne suis subject qu'à ma complexion'' (S. 74, vv. 7–8).

A verse contrasting health and sickness in sonnet 79, which was constructed as a mediation on antithetical patterns of difference and negation, illustrates the medical bipolarity of the normal and the pathological. ''Je n'escris de santé, me sentant langoureux'' (S. 79, v. 8).[104] The body of the *persona* is distinguished by the use of *langoureux*, a physiologically ambiguous term indicating someone neither sick unto death nor quite healthy. The term also represents a well-known symptom of melancholy since it denotes a body ''drayned of (naturall) moisture, deprived of vigor.''[105] Du Bellay suggests that this languishing illness had several symptoms of which the ''sick'' textual body becomes the reader. Throughout the sonnet sequence the *persona* gradually provides the model for and the interpretation of his own disorder, ascribes a variety of causes to it, and links it to several remedies.

Du Bellay's creation of pathological indices to express illness acquires a significant social connotation when one considers his personal relationships and interactions between people in the poetic text, especially his correspondence in the sonnets to friends in Rome and France. He created a representation of health and illness that was the result of, and intimately linked with, social interaction rather than being the result of the solitude and antisocial behavior characteristic of the melancholic. He produced a continual verbal elaboration of that interaction by designing a poetic discourse that he intended his peers to interpret. This has been characterized as "gestures of friendship towards friends . . . as though to improvise a fragile, invisible community."[106] Du Bellay admitted that the various types of verbal interactions found in the *Regrets* had a two-fold purpose. Firstly, they were to be regarded as no more than records or commentaries, "Pour desaigrir l'ennuy qui me tormente" (AMD. v. 80). Secondly, and more importantly, they were written to drive away idleness. "Les vers chassent de moy la molle oisiveté" (S. 14, v. 9).

The Disempowerment of Ennui and Idleness (activity-lethargy)

Melancholy was frequently considered to be a product of idleness, and exacerbated by it. Robert Burton professed that there was

> no greater cause of melancholy than idleness, ... Nothing begets it sooner, increaseth and continueth it oftener, than idleness; a disease familiar to all idle persons, an inseparable companion to such as live at ease.[107]

Moreover, the Arabic physician Rhasis affirmed that there was "no better cure [for idleness and melancholy] than business."[108]

Du Bellay demonstrated the disempowerment of idleness and the boredom of ennui by depicting their devitalizing effect on the body throughout the *Regrets* in recurring lexical patterns linking these terms with activity and inertia (*travail / paresse*), and with lack of light and restraint (*ombre /ressere*).

One example of disempowerment occurs in sonnet 58, in which Du Bellay judges a certain Le Breton at court. He criticizes his moral character and places himself on a superior moral level in comparison to Le Breton's "immoral" one. Du Bellay is satisfied by the knowledge that he is superior to Le Breton because the man is unable to master the vice of idleness.[109] The poet's moralizing conscience judges Le Breton, who excels in everything he does yet has predominant faults.

> Mais il est paresseux, & craint tant son mestier,
> Que s'il devoit jeusner, ce croy-je, un mois entier,
> Il ne travailleroit seulement un quart d'heure.
> Bref il est si poltron, pour bien le deviser.
> Que depuis quatre mois, qu'en ma chambre il demeure,
> Son ombre seulement me fait poltronniser.
>
> (*Les Regrets*, S. 58, vv. 9–14)

Treating a different aspect of idleness in Roman life, Du Bellay observes the soft idle body of "le poltron Romain" in a scathing antisocial satire. He despises the Roman for his unhealthy physique due to ''son peu d'exercice'' (S. 68, v. 8), thus acknowledging that softness and unhealthiness are signs of this leisured class.[110] This further helps to define the essential distinctness of the poet's *persona*. Du Bellay notes the consequences of idleness in Romans (''Icy l'oysiveté rend le bon vicieux'' [S. 82, v. 13]), and sharply criticized those who sheltered themselves as ''idle shut-ins'' from the cruel realities of war and suffering. They were, he wrote,

> Aveugle, sourd, & mut, plus que n'est une pierre!
> Telz sont ceulx-la (Seigneur) qu'aujourd'huy lon ressere
> Oisifz dedans leur chambre, ainsi qu'en un estuy,
> Pour durer plus long temps, & ne sentir l'ennuy,
> Que sent leur pauvre peuple accablé de la guerre.
>
> (*Les Regrets*, S. 114, vv. 4–8)

It is reasonable, and perhaps ironical as well, to find Du Bellay in sonnet 78 satirizing and condemning the seat of the Church for its idleness. In so doing he confronted the ecclesiastical position set forth during the Middle Ages that condemned melancholy as being comparable to the vice of sloth (*acedia*).

> Je te raconteray du siege de l'eglise,
> Qui fait d'oysiveté son plus riche tresor,
> Et qui dessous l'orgueil de trois couronnes d'or
> Couve l'ambition, la haine, & la feintise:
>
> (*Les Regrets*, S. 78, vv. 5–8)

Du Bellay used idleness and ennui to distinguish the categorical otherness of his poetic *persona* vis-à-vis the Roman, and to celebrate his poetic production as a way to externalize his illness. He understood poetry to be an antidote against idleness and ennui (''Les vers m'ostent l'ennuy du fascheux crediteur: / Les vers chassent de moy la molle oisiveté'' [S. 14, vv. 2, 9]), and through writing overcame the disempowerment of idleness. In so doing, he makes it clear that he was, figuratively speaking, fighting idleness with idleness. Courtiers believed that writing poetry was a senseless, idle pastime because it was unremunerated. Even Du Bellay acknowledged that it was not a particularly valuable skill.

> Et bien que Dubellay soit suffisant tesmoing,
> Combien est peu prisé le mestier de la lyre:
> Bien qu'un art sans profit ne plaise au courtisan.
>
> (*Les Regrets*, S. 11, vv. 7–9)

Yet poetry alone sustained him. He admitted that he escaped idleness by this ''leisurely kind of employment'': ''otiosaque diligentia ut vitarem torporem feriandi.''[111]

Voilà que c'est (Morel) la doulce poësie
M'accompagne par tout, sans qu'autre fantaisie
En si plaisant labeur me puisse rendre oisif.

(*Les Regrets*, S. 18, vv. 9–11)

Du Bellay's poetry served him as a form of exercise, primarily for the mind, to counter the idleness inherent in the melancholic disposition. Verses became an antidote fabricated from the prime cause of his disease. "S'il furent mon venim, le scorpion utile, / Qui sera de mon mal la seule guerison" (S. 13, vv. 13–14).[112]

Idleness and ennui are also used in the *Regrets* to focus on the body of the Romans, to denigrate their bodies, and to demonstrate the corruption within the body of the Church. Du Bellay treated idleness as a vice that must be overpowered, and which the poet's *persona* has conquered and uses to focus on the restoration of the vital nature of the body.

The Would-Be Scholar (authority and subservience)

Du Bellay also focused on the problems of the intelligent and studious man who, because of his temperament and habit, was highly susceptible to attacks of melancholia.[113] He presents the traditional studiousness and sedentary existence of the scholar in sonnet 59, in a depiction of the body of the poet's *persona*. Two distinctive signs of melancholy as a disease in the poet's *persona* are introduced: a headache and dazzled eyes.[114] Although the reader is not immediately privy to the specific disciplines of the study, it is revealed that this *persona* is an avid reader surrounded by books.[115]

Du Bellay depicts an ailing body and further develops the theme to explain the pathogenesis of the illness in terms which enable him to communicate with Pierre (who was apparently a member of the domestic staff—a barber), by providing a code for naming and classifying the indices of *ceste maladie*, yet which may exhibit misleading symptoms.[116]

Sonnet 59 reveals a gloomy poet aware that his body and its general condition are the objects of intense scrutiny. Du Bellay treats the pernicious and debilitating aspects of too much study in this poetically constructed discourse, and recommends remedies for the poetic *persona*. Pierre gives the affliction coherence by advising Du Bellay to make love instead of reading excessively.[117]

Tu ne me vois jamais (Pierre) que tu ne die
Que j'estudie trop, que je fasse l'amour,
Et que d'avoir tousjours ces livres à l'entour,
Rend les yeux eblouis, & la teste esloudie.

Mais tu ne l'entends pas: car ceste maladie
Ne me vient du trop lire, ou du trop long sejour,
Ains devoir le bureau, qui se tient chacun jour:
C'est, Pierre mon amy, le livre ou j'estudie.

(*Les Regrets*, S. 59, vv. 1–8)

The superiority of the body of the poetic *persona* as *homo melancholicus* lies in Du Bellay's privileged understanding of his condition and his power to examine the body critically, thereby reducing Pierre to a delegitimated inferior. As such, Pierre is prohibited from interpreting the mental disposition or the nature of the physical disorder as he sees it in the eyes or elsewhere on the textual body. His role is simply to occupy himself with beautifying the exterior, in order not to displease a temperament already predisposed to melancholy.

Ne m'en parle donc plus, autant que tu as cher
De me donner plaisir, & de ne me fascher:
Mais bien en ce pendant que d'une main habile
Tu me laves la barbe, & me tonds les cheveulx.

(*Les Regrets*, S. 59, vv. 9–12)

By means of this poetic discourse, Du Bellay's textual body becomes the possessor of the legitimate voice, capable of clarifying and assessing his own subject position. The courtier-poet affirms that he does indeed have a malady, but that it was caused by having to administer to the cardinal's affairs, hence: "le livre où j'estudie." In this manner, the body claims the sovereign right to frame its own identity, and resists being turned inside out by anyone but the poetic *persona* in the search for the etiology of the disorder.

A very different attitude towards disempowerment is embodied in the notion of religious hysteria. This is found in the corporeal portrayal of women in sonnets 97 and 98, in which an evil force saps the body of its strength. These two sonnets provide an interesting analogy between melancholy, the body of the poet's *persona*, and corporeal presentation of young women portrayed as *démoniaques*, especially since melancholy was also considered to be the humor of religious mania. As Lyons observes,

> Because of its heavy disposition, the melancholy mind was preoccupied with sad and frightening subjects and their symbols. The black bile produced dreams and visions connected with death and evil spirits, with night and with graveyards, and with the plants, animals or other objects that represented or embodied these.[118]

Du Bellay's morose disposition may be one reason why he related melancholy with the Roman world and dwelt on chilling descriptions of religious hysteria and demoniacal possession in the two sonnets. There is also an historical basis to this depiction based on an outbreak of religious hysteria in 1554–55, which was presumably countered by exorcism.[119] Sonnet 97, which he addressed to the physician Doulcin, assesses the inability of the "medical arts" to treat such disorders.

Doulcin, quand quelquefois je voy ces pauvres filles,
Qui ont le diable au corps, ou le semblent avoir,
D'une horrible façon corps & teste mouvoir,
Et faire ce qu'on dit de ces vieilles Sibylles:
Quand je voy les plus forts se retrouver debiles,
Voulant forcer en vain leur forcené pouvoir:
Et quand mesme j'y voy perdre tout leur sçavoir
Ceulx qui sont en vostre art tenuz des plus habiles:
Quand effroyablement escrier je les oy,
Et quand le blanc des yeux renverser je leur voy,
Tout le poil me herisse, & ne sçay plus que dire

(*Les Regrets*, S. 97, vv. 1–10)

This frightening portrait of religious hysteria developed into a vehicle for satire when Du Bellay began to portray "ces pauvres filles" as objects of a priest exorcist's attentions.

Mais quand voy un moine avec son Latin
Leur taster hault & bas le ventre & le tetin,
Ceste frayeur se passe, & suis contraint de rire.

(*Les Regrets*, S. 97, vv. 12–14)

There is almost certainly an affinity between Du Bellay's interest in producing a "stylized melancholy" in the sonnet sequence, which includes his treatment of the melancholy of the poet's *persona*, and his inclusion in the text of sonnets 97 and 98, which feature this outbreak of religious hysteria. This is especially likely given the propensity of the melancholic to be preoccupied with sad and frightening subjects, and the consequences of malady. Motifs such as these are found throughout the sonnet sequence.

The Mad Poet
(creative energy and stagnation)

Another definition of melancholy and illness appears in the *Regrets* as a corporeal phenomenon that is conjoined with a heightened awareness of the role of the poet and prose writer. Du Bellay's conception of artistic expression as madness is part of a discursive poetic practice by which men of letters were legitimated in the Renaissance. It incorporates a view of the poetic *persona* as being different from ordinary people, and therefore extraordinary. Du Bellay categorized this malady as a mode of intellectual self-definition. With it he signified what it meant to be a poet, to write "une prose en ryme, ou une ryme en prose", (S. 2 v. 10), and thus, to interpret the difference between poets' and prose writers' expertise.

> Vous dictes (Courtisans) les Poëtes sont fouls,
> Et dictes verité: mais aussi dire j'ose,
> Que telz que vous soiez, vous tenez quelque chose
> De ceste doulce humeur qui est commune à tous.
> Mais celle-la (Messieurs) qui domine sur vous,
> En autres actions diversement s'expose:
> Nous sommes fouls en rime, & vous l'estes en prose:
> C'est la seul difference qi'est entre vous & nous.
>
> (*Les Regrets*, S. 149 vv. 1–8)

Du Bellay also used *ceste doulce humeur* to establish the body as a valued object and to valorize the elite position of the Renaissance courtier-poet. Verses such as ''J'ay le corps maladif / Je suis né pour la Muse, on me fait mesnager'' (S. 39 vv. 12–13), and ''je travaille mon corps d'un indigne exercice'' (S. 45 v. 13), affirm the exclusivity of the textual body. When Du Bellay interprets a condition of disorder in the ''corps maladif'' of the poet's *persona*, and denotes illness as a divine gift ''commune à tous,'' he is assuming their social function. He realizes that the afflictions will be interpreted in the Renaissance world of *Literati* as representing valid knowledge of their extraordinary position in society.

These brief portraits of melancholia and its physical aspects illustrate that a ''stylized melancholy'' is present in the *Regrets* as a discourse engaged in by the textual body. Insofar as this ''illness'' is developed in the course of Du Bellay's sojourn in Rome, it becomes, in the sonnet sequence, a specific stylistic problem that requires him to interpret, analyze, and to provide some kind of answer regarding its etiology, and to develop an artistic concern for its cure. As such, the discourse on melancholia is used as a means of examining the body and its vice or affectation. As an illness, it is often amplified by the poet into the proportions of an obsession, and humoral imbalance, most particularly visible in the preoccupation with excessive self-pity, and in the association of intelligence with poetic inspiration. The discourse on melancholia frequently becomes a vehicle for satire or, in lesser examples, an object of interest and amazement to the poet. However, the use of a new poetic form in the *Regrets*, which included the use of a ''stylized melancholy,'' and with which the poet declared: ''Moy, qui suis malheureux, je plaindray mon malheur'' (S. 5, v. 14), and ''Je ne chante (Magny) je pleure mes ennuys'' (S. 12, v. 5), is not presented without preoccupation on the part of the poet. Du Bellay was concerned that writing this new type of poetry would be poorly received and therefore damage his reputation. identity of his subjects for more clarity.

Chapter III
Religious Discourse:
The *physiologie chrestienne*

The desire to explore and delineate the boundaries of Christian physiology, which belongs to a long tradition of humanist debate in Europe over man's place in the universe, is evident in the works of numerous French poets during the periods of religious turmoil in the Reformation; poetic representations of Catholic and Huguenot bodies commonly appear in texts of polemical poetry.[120]

Pastor Simon Goulart of Geneva, a ''preeminent''[121] compiler and critical commentator of historical and political writings and authors during the later part of the sixteenth century, stressed the importance of gaining knowledge of man's Christian physiology. Doing so, he said,

> is worthy of all Christians, most profitable, and necessarie for Theologians, and in the Bookes of the ancient Doctors; . . . there are scattered fragments full of singular instruction . . . to the end to elevate our minds, (as it were by degrees) to the Creator.
>
> It remaineth that some one take the paine to gather this Phisiologie out of the bookes of the Prophets and Apostles, as also from other learned persons that came after them.[122]

Goulart believed that exploring and interpreting this physiology required a methodological approach and diligent scrutiny of the properties of the body. He asserted that this interpretation should be effected systematically through faith and careful retrieval (''gathering'') and cataloguing widely dispersed and diversified writings from both ancient and modern times. Goulart examined the works of one of these writers, Protestant poet Guillaume De Saluste Sieur Du Bartas, whose approach to the question compared with his. The pastor focused on the *physiologie chrestienne* in his learned summaries of the ''Sixth Day'' and ''Seventh Day'' of Du Bartas' *Première semaine*, and furnished clear evidence of the poet's intention to delineate such a physiology. He perceived the ''Seventh Day'' as a poem in which the

> poet proposeth or setteth downe the foundations of a Christian physiologie, teaching the Readers to consider the Creatures of God with an eye purified by faith.[123]

This chapter is intended to supplement Goulart's commentary on the *physiologie chrestienne* during the French Reformation and further develop the theme by examining the political poetry of two of Du Bartas' contemporaries, the Catholic poet Pierre de Ronsard (the *Discours des Misères*, the *Continuation*, and the *Remonstrance*), and the Protestant poet Agrippa D'Aubigné (*Les Tragiques*).[124] Their definitions and interpretations of this physiology differed markedly from Goulart's and Du Bartas' and from each other's.

I examine their adherence to a subjective perspective of physiology in how they addressed certain concepts of foreignness and strangeness, the problems of the self and of difference, authority and legitimacy in their representations, and the resulting ontological instability of the body in their polemical poetry.

These poetic texts describe events in the French civil wars and reflect profound and complex changes that swept Europe at the dissolution of a united Christendom. This schism resulted in two Christian bodies—Catholic and Protestant—that viewed each other as being fundamentally different. The Protestants' *foi estrange* provided a radically new historical and theological experience. Poets attempted to discover and authenticate factual differences between the two faiths that varied according to their own religious perspective. They did so by recording these dissimilarities in terms such as strangeness, aberrations, physical peculiarities, nonconformity, eccentric behavior, and foreignness, often relating them to the body. One of their principal concerns (and mine) pertained to problems of analyzing and representing the lines of demarcation between a bipartite Christian physiology.

Ronsard and D'Aubigné both tried to involve the reader in defining and interpreting a Christian physiology, and each focused on the human body as it functions as referential marker and narrative for social and religious critique. Both poets viewed the body as the locus for representing its fragile composition in various forms and as the ground on which to contest Protestant and Catholic social and religious conflicts. They reconfigured literal and figurative meanings of the human body; each encouraged a reexamination of the association between that complex entity and social and religious attitudes. The construction of a Catholic-Protestant duality in these exemplary poems illustrates the infinite distance that separates the two bodies and underscores their fundamentally different corporeality. This duality engendered endless polemics in Reformation literature.

Protestant Martyrology

At the core of D'Aubigné's *Les Tragiques* is the concept of the Protestant body as a matrix for representing consensual violence, a violence that emanates from ''outside'' agents of ''otherness,'' i.e. Catholics. He poignantly portrays the drama of this body unjustly incarcerated, persecuted and martyred for religious reasons. Protestants are ''tragic ones'' in a ''felicitous'' drama, tormented heroes and heroines subjected to violence and suffering essential for martyrdom's ironic triumph.[125]

Martyred Protestant bodies differed from Catholic ones, according to D'Aubigné, because they bore scars of torture that inscribed themselves figuratively on the living. Whatever the theological implications of martyrdom, he deliberately venerated the body, portraying it as a mechanism for suffering through martyr imagery, and consequently reified it as a locus of martyrological worship. Martyrs were extreme examples of what all good Christians should aspire to: the mortification of the flesh. *Vengeances* (book six of *Les Tragiques*) details the ''true'' Christian's yearning for martyrdom.[126]

> Venez donc pauvreté, faim, fuittes et blessures,
> Bannissements, prison, proscriptions, injures;
> Vienne l'heureuse mort, gage pour tout jamais
> De la fin de la guerre et de la douce paix!
> Fuyez triomphes vains, la richesse et la gloire,
> Plaisirs, prosperité, insolente victoire,
> O pieges dangereuses et signes evidens
> Des tenebres, du ver, et grincement de dents!
>
> (*Vengeances*, vv. 733–740)

D'Aubigné described the corporeal stance of Catholics, who represented evil forces, as *l'atheiste affligeant* rather than as a form of aberrant Christianity. Their deserved punishment delighted him, just as the martyrdom of his fellow Protestant—*le chrestien affligé*—elicited his admiration. He invites the reader to compare both from a Protestant perspective.

> Nous sommes plein de sang, l'un en perd, l'autre en tire
> L'un est persecuteur, l'autre endure martyre:
> Regardez qui reçoit ou qui donne le coup.
> Ne criez sur l'agneau quand vous criez au loup.
>
> (*Les Fers*, vv. 1545–48)

One of the most fundamental issues D'Aubigné discoursed upon was how a Protestant's body differed from that of a Catholic. He used poetic symmetry to portray this dual sense of Christian physiology, and illustrated several differences by using words that play upon dissimilarities (e.g., *perd*, *tire*, *persecuteur* and *martyre*). He contrasted Christian lambs and Catholic wolves in the antithetical use of moral references, depicting the line of demarcation between the two as being substantially that of opressed Christians and atheist persecutors.

The opening lines of the fourth book of *Les Tragiques*, *Les Feux*, deal with the relationship between martyrs, martyrology and the text. D'Aubigné glorifies the agonies of Protestant martyrs, of whom only ashes remained to be scattered to the winds (*Les Feux*, vv. 67–72). *Les Tragiques* is a virtual of portrait gallery that exhibits inspirational exempla and reveals that its predominant structural principle is to provide a lasting *tableau* of the civil wars. The word *tableau* (*Les Feux*, v. 22), referring to the text, provides a unifying frame and symbol of the martyr.

Protestants disdained Catholic saints and disapproved of fragmenting saints' bodies into relics for distribution to churches and holy sites.[127] Clearly, the bodies of Protestant martyrs could not be so employed. However, D'Aubigné demonstrated that Protestant martyrs' bodies could be immortalized by displaying them in the poetic text. He replaced the customary relic crucial to martyr worship with a recuperated textual body and intermingled it with a demonstration of his authorial self-awareness, insisting that he would use his own voice (but with divine inspiration) to revivify martyrs.

> Condui mon oeuvre, ô Dieu! à ton nom, donne moy
> Qu'entre tant de martyrs, champions de la foy,
> De chasque sexe, estat ou aage, à ton sainct temple
> Je puisse consacrer un tableau pour exemple
>
> (*Les Feux*, vv. 19–22)

D'Aubigné's martyrological rhetoric mingles obscurity and clarity; in any case, martyrs who die in the *laide nuict* must be viewed. His text, which he considered to be an ideal way to reveal the unseen, provided the means for achieving that recognition, replacing—or rather functioning as—the traditional relic, thus assuring future generations access to it. Catharine Randall Coates suggests that this type of text may serve "in some sense like a reliquary, in that it carefully houses the precious remnants of the martyr's existence, his speech and last acts."[128] The following passage illustrates D'Aubigné's intention to lift the veil of obscurity and reconstruct visually a new textual body of the martyr.

> O bien-heureux celuy qui, quand l'homme le tue,
> Arrache de l'erreur tant d'esprits par sa veuë,
> Qui monstre les thresors et graces de son Dieu,
> Qui butine en mourant tant d'esprits au milieu

Des spectateurs esleus: telle mort est suivie
Presque tousjours du gain de mainte belle vie.
Mais les martyrs ont eu moins de contentement
De qui la laide nuict cache le beau tourment:
Non que l'ambition y soit quelque salaire,
Le salaire est en Dieu à qui la nuict est claire;
Pourtant beau l'instrument de qui l'exemple sert
A gaigner en mourant la brebis qui se perd.
Je ne t'oublieray pas, ô ame bien-heureuse!
Je tireray ton nom de la nuict tenebreuse;
Ton martyre secret, ton exemple caché
Sera par mes escrits des ombres arraché.

(*Les Feux*, vv. 981–996)

This passage in which D'Aubigné promotes Protestantism by authenticating the words of the poem (*mes escrits*) as a relic, and the text as a reliquary, is a significant commentary on the importance of the text as instrument in Renaissance France. He again reveals that the poem's predominant structural principle is to validate and protect the Protestant cause.

Protestant Tyrants and Catholic Victims

Most of Ronsard's political poems, particularly the *Continuation*, express a similar desire to provide an historical document that will permit future generations to understand the deserved misfortunes of those who rebel against their (Catholic) rulers. Ronsard and D'Aubigné had comparable desires for personal recognition, and they both wanted to establish the framework of a Christian physiology. Ronsard does this by superimposing Catholic rather than Protestant discourse in the poetic text.

Ce pendant pren la plume, & d'un stile endurci
Contre le trait des ans, engrave tout ceci,
A fin que nos nepveux puissent un jour cognoistre
Que l'homme est malheureux qui se prend à son maistre.

(*Continuation*, vv. 441–444)

Ronsard used techniques similar to D'Aubigné to distort and therefore damn Protestant physiology. Obviously, he interpreted the Protestant obsession with emulating martyrs in an entirely different manner. His poems redefine Protestant martyrs as tyrants and create tension between the identities of genuine and counterfeit martyrs. He creates a textual body of the Protestant martyr that shows him to be at once a hypocritical impostor, artificial, delusory, and fraudulent. Ronsard represented the Catholic (himself) as "un homme qui mesprise / vos songes contrefais" (*Continuation*, vv. 163–4), while he viewed Protestants as *nouveaux*

Tyrans led by rhetoricians who "preschent autrement qu'ils ont dedans les coeurs" (*Continuation*, v. 182), and by preachers "Ayant de soubs un raistre une espée au costé," (*Continuation*, v. 148).

The poet accomplishes his portrayal of Protestant physiology largely by superimposing objects on the body that distort its exterior, i.e., *un raistre*, *une espée*. He undermines the image of Protestants submitting voluntarily to torture by portraying them as bearing arms rather than patiently suffering martyrdom; their bodies are "toujours de corcelets armez" (*Continuation*, v. 86).

Ha que vous estes loing de nos premiers docteurs,
Qui sans craindre la mort ny les persecuteurs,
Alloient de leur bon gré aux plus cruels suplices,
Sans envoyer pour eux je ne scay quels novices.

(*Continuation*, vv. 197–200)

Ronsard also records differences between Catholic and Protestant bodies in recurring images that illustrate his belief that the Catholic possesses a victim's body. This is exemplified by his reference to the body of France as a symbol of the Catholic state cruelly and despotically treated by Protestant tyrants and brigands.

Mais ces nouveaux Tyrans qui la France ont pillée,
Vollée, assassinée, à force despouillée,
Et de cent mille coups le corps luy ont batu,
(Comme si brigandage estoit une vertu)

(*Continuation*, vv. 23–26)

Equally striking are the lines in which he condemns Protestants for crimes that threaten France's body politic. He portrays the corporeal fury of Huguenot vandalism and denounces their postures and their fraudulent faith (Fig. 3.1., "Horribles cruautez des Huguenots en France").

Or eux se vantant seuls les vrais enfans de Dieu,
En la dextre ont le glaive, & en l'autre le feu,
Et comme furieux qui frappent & enragent,
Vollent les temples saincts, & les villes sacagent.
Et quoy! bruler maisons, piller & brigander,
Tuer, assassiner, par force commander,
N'obeir plus aux Roys, amasser des armées,
Appellez vous cela Eglises reformées?

(*Discours*, vv. 41–48)

Ronsard makes a similar point in the *Remonstrance*, in which he portrays himself as the victim of inhuman cruelties at the hands of Huguenot tyrants.

Horribles cruautez des Huguenotz en France.

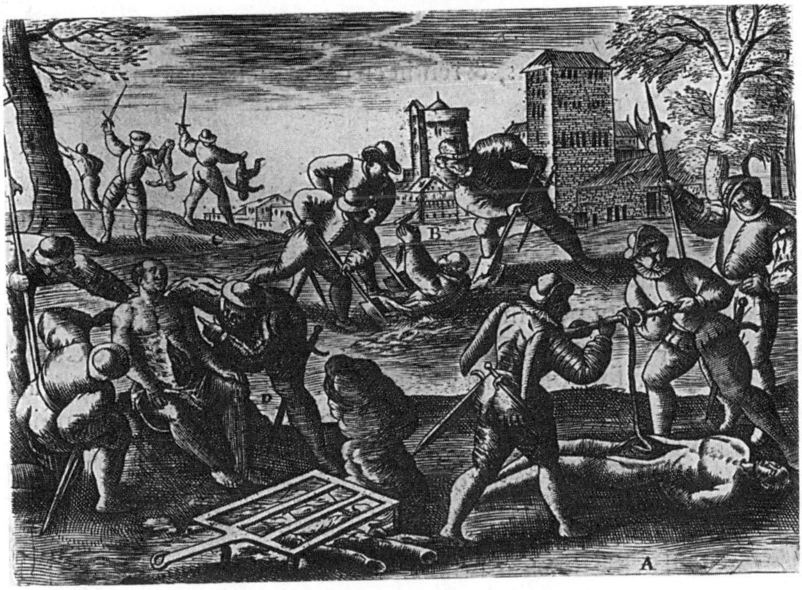

Ces tyrans inſenſeZ n'eſtants iamais contents;
Jnuentent tous les iours autres nouueaux torments;
A leur ardant courroux ne ſuffit nulle paine:
Jlz s'eſgaient à voir ſouffrir cruelle mort.
Aux pauures innocents, qu'ilZ font mourir à tort,
Montrant par tel tourments leur tant mortelle haine.

G Dv

Figure 3.1 "Horribles cruautez des Huguenots en France," Richard Verstegen, from *Theatre des cruautez des hereticques de nostre temps*, Anvers, A. Hubert, 1607. (Photo: By Permission of the Folger Shakespeare Library.)

Je sçay qu'ils sont cruels & tirans inhumains:
N'agueres le bon Dieu me sauva de leurs mains,
Apres m'avoir tiré cinq coups de harquebuse:

(*Remonstrance*, vv. 545–47)

"Je pense encore voir un monstrueux geant,"

(*Les Tragiques*, *Misères*, v. 135)

Analogous to Ronsard's image of Catholic France's battered and assassinated body politic is D'Aubigné's depiction of the victimized nation as having the diseased, disordered and deteriorating body of a *monstrueux geant*. This metaphorical figure embodies the Protestant-Catholic struggle in national terms. D'Aubigné's image of this giant begins as a portrait of France as an afflicted mother of two, one Catholic and the other Protestant, but his corporeal vocabulary transforms it into something quite different and of particular interest.[129] He recognized this giant as being an extraordinary public sign, or message, to the people of France. Consequently, he did not inquire into its properties and qualities, or treat it as an "unnatural phenomenon" that required a scientific explanation. He sternly advised his countrymen to pay heed to the giant's message: "Vous n'estes spectateurs, vous estes personnages:" (*Misères*, v. 170).

D'Aubigné focused on the physiological functions of this *corps divisé* rather than on its anatomy. He offered insights into essential, but hidden, workings of its physical nature, and in doing so revealed much about sixteenth century medical theories. His description contains abundant physiological details of a diseased body, and is thus a rich source of information about the way in which illness was then recognized and understood. He subscribed to the Greek medical theory that disease affected the body's temperament, and to the belief that there were four distinctive bodily fluids or "humors"—blood, phlegm, bile (or choler), and black bile (or melancholy)—that were indispensable to the body's physiological functions.[130] He used numerous images of corporeality to describe the giant's ordeal and to register the effects of illnesses and disease on its figure, and attributes them to religious conflict. D'Aubigné identified certain conditions in terms of external symptoms that he conceptualized within the framework of the complexion theory. He depicts the giant's failing condition in the following verses in which he cites changes in the blood that indicate the presence of biles (choler) and phlegm, thus substantiating the existence of humoral imbalances.

Son corps est combatu, à soi-mesme contraire:
Le sang pur ha le moins, le flegme et la colere
Rendant le sang non sang: . . .

. . .
La masse degenere en la melancholie;
Ce vieil corps tout infect, plein de sa discrasie,
Hydropique, fait l'eau, si bien que ce geant
Qui alloit de ses nerfs ses voisins outrageant,
Aussi foible que grand n'enfle plus que son ventre.

(*Misères*, vv. 141–149)

D'Aubigné only analyzed diseases that affected the entire body, doing so according to their complexional attributes. He classified dropsy (*hydropique*) as wet and dyscrasia (*discrasie*) as dry; the former was a morbid condition, the latter a wasting disease that caused an ill complexion or appearance.[131] Afflictions eroded the giant's corporeal identity as a figure of immense proportions to one depicted by D'Aubigné as a degenerating mass of *melancholie*.[132]

The poet also examined various nutritive functions and malfunctions of this impaired body. He recognized that blood was important to the body's nutrition; ingested food was transformed into chyle in the stomach and blood in the liver and diffused throughout the body. He observed that these functions were impaired in the diseased and impotent body of France, and linked them to the theme of a "topsy-turvy" world in which the giant was transformed into a horrible beast.

Ce ventre dans lequel tout se tire, tout entre,
Ce faux dispensateur des communs excremens
N'envoye plus aux bords les justes alimens:
Des jambes et des bras les os sont sans moelle.
Il ne va plus en haut pour nourir la cervelle
Qu'un chime venimeux dont le cerveau est nourri
Ce grand geant changé en une horrible beste
A sur ce vaste corps une petite teste,
Deux bras foibles pendans, des-ja secs, des-ja morts,
Impuissans de nourrir et defendre le corps;
Les jambes sans pouvoir porter leur masse lourde
Et à gauche et à droit font porter une bourde.

(*Misères*, vv. 150–162)

A singular paradigm of physical evil that materializes most often in dehumanized and bestialized forms emerges from the various images of the victimized body in both poets' work. D'Aubigné links this evil to the parallel theme of man's inhumanity to man that appears as a complicated physiological pattern notable in his expressions *horrible beste* and *monstrueux geant*. It also appears in his antithetical use of moral references such as Christian lambs and Catholic wolves. Conversely, this theme is found in Ronsard's *tirans inhumains* and *changé de couleur & de teint*.

A striking aspect of this polemical poetry is that these diametrically opposed poets placed remarkably similar emphasis on the theme of man's dehumanization and bestialization. Each incorporated powerful symbols of corporeal transmutations and disassemblage in his poetic text: the metamorphosis of a human body (albeit that of a giant) into a monstrous beast with a shrunken head and crippled arms and legs, or into inhuman tyrants changing cloaks and appearance (examined below).[133] These transformations, which created a new textual body upon which both poets superimposed their beliefs and concepts of reality through poetic discourse, formed extensive frames of reference that reached far beyond the merely physiological. They stressed the significance of the comportment defining Catholic and Protestant bodies and created models of physical evil common to both, not only in acts of violence but in a wider theological interpretation that equates the body with sin. Moreover, there is considerable iconographic support for the poetic convention of creating a new textual body by incorporating animal imagery (Fig. 3.2., Huguenots portrayed as apes, considered as symbols of profanity). This concentration on a new textual body, which is especially useful in analyzing D'Aubigné's treatment of Henry III's body, is studied in greater detail below.

However, as we move from the analysis of the textual tradition of bestialization and dehumanization to foreignness, (*estrangeté*), we find a slightly different dimension of the theme of corporeal deviations in Ronsard's Catholic poems as he focuses on depicting the Protestant as being physically aberrant.

Ronsard and the Protestant as Enemy

Ronsard's *Discours* and *Continuation* characterize the Protestant as an enemy whose body is altered forever by the effects of this radically new *foi estrange*. He used this concept of *estrange*, which designated foreignness and difference, to expose and reinforce dissimilarities between Protestants and Catholics. Protestants (e.g., Huguenots, Lutherans, Zwinglians, and Calvinists) followed "L'erreur d'un estranger."

> Faittes moy voir quelqu'un qui ait changé
> Apres avoir suivy vostre belle folie?
> J'en voy qui ont changé de couleur & de teint,
>
> Hydeux en barbe longue, & en visage feint,
> Qui sont plus que devant tristes, mornes & palles,
> Comme Oreste agité des fureurs infernalles.
>
> (*Continuation*, vv. 259–64)

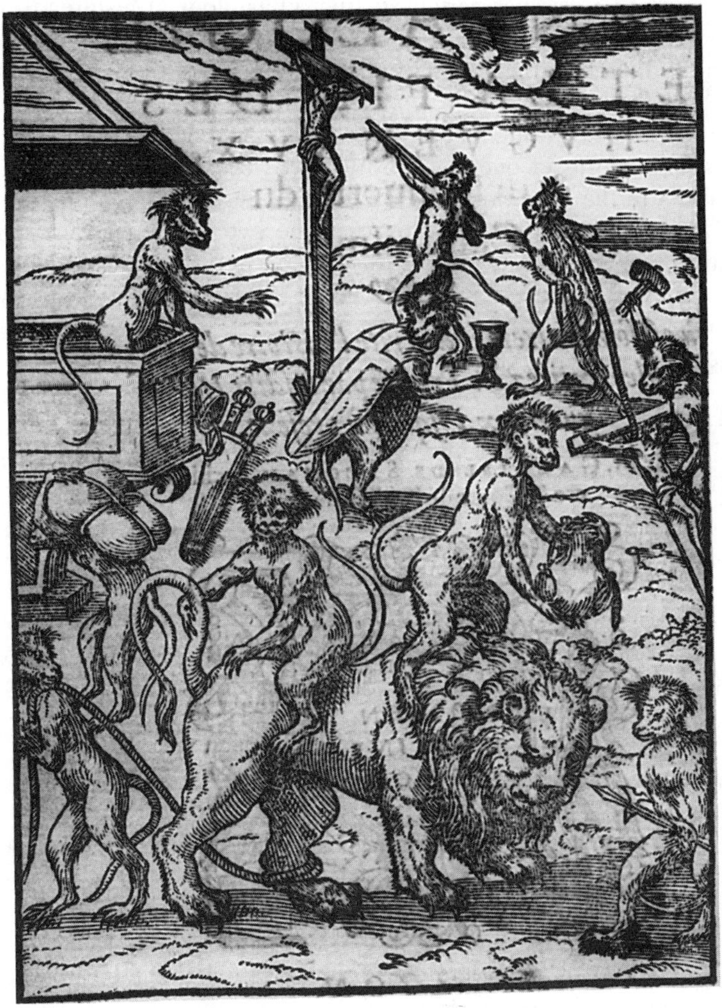

EZECHIEL XXIX.

Je t'ay liuré aux bestes de la terre pour estre deuoré.

Figure 3.2 Huguenots portrayed as apes, Gabriel de Saconay, from *Genealogie et la Fin des Huguenaux*, Lyon, B. Rigaud, 1573. (Photo: Courtesy of The Newberry Library, Chicago.)

In these verses he ascribes certain distinct physiological features to Protestants and suggests that they may be interpreted through the art of physiognomy, which was then an important component of an aristocratic education.[134]

Ronsard affirms throughout the *Discours* that vice deforms the body; "Il nous faut confesser que le vice diforme," (*Discours*, v. 7). He vividly portrays this in the *Continuation*, in which Protestants are addressed in the "vous" form to denote the gulf between the two groups and to stigmatize Protestants as being diseased and disfigured. Ronsard's diatribe was also aimed at the aging Calvin, who had gained the reputation in France of a *martyr glorieux* (v. 201).

> Vous ressemblés à ceux que les fiebvres incensent
> . . .
> Le peuple qui vous suit est tout empoisonné
> Il a tant le cerveau de sectes estonné
> Que toute la Rubarbe & toute l'Anticyre
> Ne lui scauroient garir sa fiebvre qui empire;
> Car tant s'en faut helas! qu'on la puisse garir,
> Que son mal le contente, & luy plaist d'en mourir.
>
> (*Continuation*, vv. 179, 209–214)

The etiology of the Protestant body's menacing disease is the renunciation of "La foy de ses ayeulz pour en prendre une estrange" (*Discours*, v. 40). Ronsard interprets *fiebvres* (diseases suffered by Protestants) as being punitive phenomena caused by transgressions; he affixes their exegesis as a sign of merited and divine retribution. In this sense, the altered and abnormal comportment caused by these *fiebvres* become visible signs of Protestant corruption and guilt.

Ronsard paints a poetic panorama of symptoms that provides an excellent insight into the "abnormalities" of the Protestant body. This is illustrated in the *Remonstrance*, which refers to a Protestant's disease as *vostre contagion* (v. 229), thus revealing its communicability. Ronsard asserts that no medicinal elixirs or antidotes are available to infected Protestants. Even administering massive doses of widely recommended remedies such as *rubarbe* and *l'Anticyre* to cure "fevers" or madness would be ineffective.[135] They may only be cured and their diseased and poisoned bodies purified by admitting their errors, renouncing the *foi estrange*, undergoing penance, and returning to "La foy de ses ayeulz" ("the belief of his forebearers"): the true Roman Catholic faith.

Ronsard reaffirmed his Catholic viewpoint in the final verse quoted above: "Que son mal le contente, & luy plaist d'en mourir." Death is the implicit fate of diseased Protestants (including Calvin) who refuse to confess their errors and repent. But the verse contains something even more fundamental: Ronsard's explicit acknowledgment, which he had previously denied (*Continuation*, vv. 197–200), of the Protestants' status as martyrs in which the body plays a prominent role. Unwittingly perhaps, he participated in defining the martyr. The image of the body in the verse is very clearly that of a martyr; it depicts two kinds of bodily experiences prerequisite to martyr status. First, the reference to disease (*mal*) records the martyrs ordeal by providing a visible manifestation of their degradation and by revealing the circumstances of their suffering. Ronsard links this disease to the Protestants' complacency ("Que son mal le contente"), and provides evidence of their willingness to suffer for a cause. Second, their deaths become a statement of eternal life. Surrendering to a hostile power and voluntarily accepting death rather than renounce one's beliefs may be interpreted as a confirmation of martyrdom. Clearly, the disease Ronsard meant as punishment must also be interpreted as a confirmation of martyrdom. This example, however, should not be considered typical of Ronsard. He was obsessed elsewhere in his work with invalidating the Protestants' martyrological status by creating tension between them and legitimate martyrs. His political poems are filled with forceful denunciations of heretical Protestants: "Le Huguenot mutin, l'heretique mechant," tyrants and brigands. The *Discours des Misères et autres pièces politiques* fails to restore the Protestant body to Catholicism; it merely observes, confirms and condemns it. D'Aubigné's *Les Tragiques* preserves a painful recognition of the tortured and martyred Protestant body and condemns the Catholic as fraudulent.

Catholic and Protestant bodies often coexist in these works, in which mutually bitter denunciations apparently had no effect on the other except to provoke vehement retorts. The perception each poet had about the "body" of the opposing faith was derived from deeply-held religious convictions and was manifested largely by visual vocabulary. They directed this at readers who interpreted what they read in terms relative to their respective beliefs. Catholics recognized the Protestants' alien customs and peculiar physical appearance, and designate him as the "others," while they believed that they represented the legitimate body of the true faith. Similarly, Protestants identified Catholics as atheist persecutors while identifying themselves with the first Christians, as true martyrs. Each group challenged the authority of the body of the other. D'Aubigné accused Catholics (particularly the royal family) of being atheists, and repeatedly denounced their murderous and enemy hands: *la main ennemie* (*Misères*, v. 1033), *sanglantes mains* (*Les Feux*, v. 1015), *mains impures* (*Princes*, v. 418). Ronsard repudiated Protestant accusations of atheism in verses that reinforced his view of Protestant bodies as being illegitimate inhabitants of their *pays natal* and as unnatural *monstres de l'Eglise* who suffered from delusions (a reference to their *songes contrefais*). Ronsard was, in his own way, a reformer intent upon destroying the ideal of the Protestant martyr created by the Reformers.

Adonq je respondi: apellés vous Athée
La personne qui point n'a de son coeur ostée
La foy de ses ayeux ? qui ne trouble les loix
De son pays natal, les peuples ny les Roys?
Apellés vous Athée, un homme qui mesprise
Vos songes contrefais, les monstres de l'Eglise?
Qui croit en un seul Dieu, qui croit au sainct Esprit
Qui croit de tout son coeur au sauveur Jesuschrist?
Apellés vous Athée un homme qui deteste
Et vous & vos erreurs comme infernale peste?

(*Continuation*, vv. 159–168)

Conversely, D'Aubigné denounced poets who supported the Catholic cause as "vos rhymeurs hypocrites / Desguisez, ont changé tant de phrases escrites" (*Princes*, vv. 429–30). He dismissed their work as *fables mensongeres* (*Princes*, v. 434) while legitimizing his text, thereby authenticating the body of the Protestant martyr as the rightful heir to the kingdom of God.

Tu es né legitimement,
Dieu mesme a donné l'argument,
Je ne te donne qu'à l'Eglise
Tu as pour support l'equité
Pour loyer l'immortalité

(*Préface*, vv. 409–414)

Royal Bodies of Power: A Topsy-Turvy World

The centrality of the image of legitimacy in D'Aubigné's poetry is apparent, and prominent in his examination of royal bodies and in his numerous invalidations of their corporeal identities. Most striking is his examination of physiological degeneracy in the form of bodily deviations, deceptions, and sexual perversions permeating the decadent Catholic court of Henry III, Catherine de Medici and the Mignons. Richard Regosin observes that the king symbolized "the disorder of the 'monde à l'envers,' "; his "femininity and homosexuality, as perversions of nature, stamp[ed] him as a monster, outside the bounds of the natural."[136] D'Aubigné used the themes of bestiality and dehumanization to illustrate this degeneracy. He reasoned that mankind lost its humanity by reverting to the animal state; "les loups et les renards et les bestes sauvages tienent place d'humains" (*Misères*, vv. 325–26). The poet frequently employed animal or monster terminology to incarnate these figures in binary relationships of opposition and contradiction.

After generalizing on the animalistic nature of man, D'Aubigné depicted Henry III and the Mignons as sodomites and hermaphrodites, creatures of contradictory sexual identities. He thereby provided a more detailed example of the body in the topos of the disordered world. The king and his court provided the poet with an epistemological structure based on a fundamental biological metaphor for expressing conflict. This metaphor ultimately became a significant emblem of the decadence of the age. D'Aubigné's interest in hermaphroditism illustrates his thorough but arcane knowledge of related philosophical, religious and poetic texts. He may have drawn inspiration from several contemporary sources such as Ambroise Paré's medical works and his treatise on bizarre creatures entitled *Des monstres et prodiges* (1573). Numerous writers accused Henry and royal courtiers of sodomy. Thomas Artus' satire on the court, *L'Isle des hermaphrodites* (1605), (Fig. 3.3., ''Les Hermaphrodites''), portrays the bisexuality of the king and his Mignons, as does Henri Estienne's *Apologie pour Hérodote: Satire de la société au XVIe siècle* (1566).[137]

The eponymous myth of Hermaphrodites was prominent in classical literature (e.g. Ovid and Plato), and was also a significant artistic theme prior to and during the Renaissance. That D'Aubigné was aware of at least certain aspects of the mythical nature of the subject is indicated by his reference to Sardanapalus,[138] yet he largely ignored the classical origins of this myth; both Ovid and Plato may have influenced his conception of the hermaphrodite, but neither dominates his representations. Instead, D'Aubigné focuses one dimensionally on the ambivalent sexual significance of the hermaphrodite, polemicizing a basic aspect of its paradox and underscoring the difference between Henry III and *de vraix Rois.* He equates hermaphrodites with transvestism and homosexuality, and characterizes the hermaphroditic king and his courtiers as symbols of weakness, corruption, and evil.

Qui, philosophe et Roy, regne par la science,
Et n'est fait impuissant par sa grande puissance!
    Ceux-là regnent vraiment, ceux-là sont de vrais Rois
Qui sur leurs passions establissent des loix,
Qui regnent sur eux mesme, et d'une ame constante
Domptent l'ambition volage et impuissante:
Non les hermaphrodits, monstres effeminez,
Corrompus, bourdeliers, et qui estoyent mieux nez
Pour valets des putains que seigneurs sur les hommes,
Non les monstres du siecle et du temps où nous sommes;
Non pas ceux qui sous l'or, sous le pourpre royal,

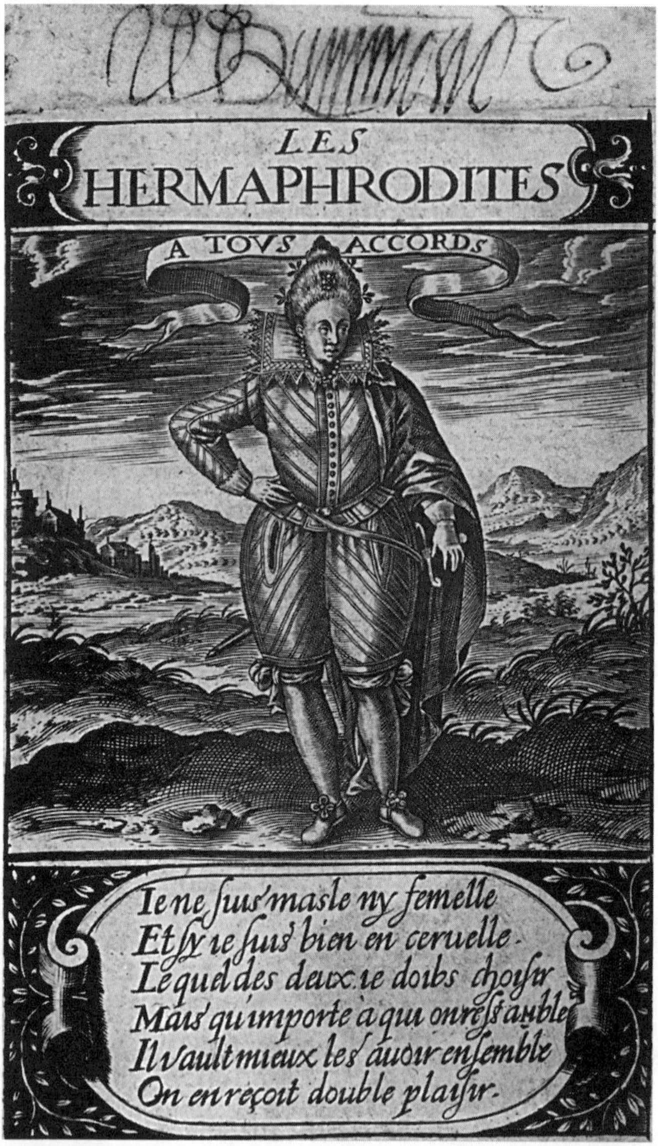
LES
HERMAPHRODITES
A TOVS ACCORDS
Ie ne suis masle ny femelle
Et sy ie suis bien en ceruelle.
Lequel des deux ie doibs choysir
Mais qu'importe à qui on ressamble
Il vault mieux les auoir ensemble
On en reçoit double plaisir.

Figure 3.3 Portrait of Henri III, title page and six lines of verse from Thomas Artus. *Les hermaphrodites*, n.p., 1605?. (Photo: By Permission of The Folger Shakespeare Library.)

> Couvent la lascheté, un penser desloyal,
> La trahison des bons, un mespris de la charge
> Que sur le dos d'un Roy un bon peuple descharge:
>
> (*Princes*, vv. 661–674)

D'Aubigné was inspired by more than creative poetic ambition in his investigation and condemnation of female behavioral characteristics such as effeminacy, passivity and weakness—*effeminez* and *lascheté*—when manifested in a male subject. He reflected contemporary medical views on sexuality in several ways and, although he was more strongly misogynistic than Paré, supported Paré's interpretation of the biological differences of the sexes as opposites, with the male being the active principle and the female the passive.[139] D'Aubigné's poetic strategy concerning Henry's ambiguous gender was to obscure deliberately the king's gender and treat him simply as a human subject who, disguised as a female, deviates from the sexual norm.

This iconography of the monarch encourages the reader to question not only the king-subject relationship in French society, but also the relationship between power, authority and sexuality implicit in the conventions of kingship. D'Aubigné used the motif of skepticism to reintroduce animal terminology and to characterize and present Henry III physically as *ce doubteux animal* (*Princes*, v. 777). He reinforces this perplexing image and creates ambiguous subject positions for the monarch's body and his entourage by referring the tensions of mistaken gender identity to the reader. He does this by declaring that there is "en la place d'un Roy, une putain fardée" (*Princes*, v. 784) whose courtiers manifest "le geste effeminé, l'oeil d'un Sardanapale" (*Princes*, v. 776).[140]

This moral indictment of royal behavior reveals another rhetorical strategy D'Aubigné used to create poetically a crisis of representation in which the king's body reflected no stable biological distinction between male or female. His body is imagined and shaped through discursive categories that problematize male and female. This allows the poet to comment upon sexuality in paradoxical shifts of representation and also to discuss the social structure and behavior of the sixteenth-century court. Describing the spectacle at a court masquerade ball, D'Aubigné provides a representation of Henry III that compares an ideal *Roy* to its parody, the *putain fardée*. He reinforces that image in a similar verse in which he postulates on the figure's dual gender : *un Roy femme* or *un homme Reyne*. The poet skilfully evokes the spectacle of Henry's appearance at the ball by portraying his arrival attired

De cordons emperlez sa chevelure plein,
Sous un bonnet sans bord fait à l'italienne,
Faisoit deux arcs voutez; son menton pinceté,
Son visage de blanc et de rouge empasté,
Son chef tout empoudré nous monstrerent ridée,
En la place d'un Roy, une putain fardee.
Pensez quel beau spectacle, et comm' il fit bon voir
Ce prince avec un busc, un corps de satin noir
Couppé à l'espagnolle, où, des dechicquetures,
Sortoyent des passements et des blanches tireures;
Et, affin que l'habit s'entresuivist de rang,
Il monstroit des manchons gauffrez de satin blanc,
D'autres manches encor qui s'estendoyent fendues,
Et puis jusques aux pieds d'autres manches perdues.
Pour nouveau parement il porta tout ce jour
Cet habit monstrueux, pareil à son amour:
Si qu'au premier bord chacun estoit en peine
S'il voyait un Roy femme ou bien un homme Reyne.

(*Princes*, vv. 779–796)

Satirizing Henry's womanish appearance was essentially a theatrical game for D'Aubigné, one intended both to amuse and to confuse the reader as spectator, and to demonstrate that one could not see or know the king's body because its proper proportions were disguised by his *habit monstrueux*. Nevertheless, the poet used the "spectacle" to reinforce his opinion that effeminacy in a male is a reprehensible transgression of proper gender behavior, even though his feminine model of the king does have inevitable blind spots and distortions.[141] Yet the verses describing the court ball contain an important confirmation regarding D'Aubigné's recognition of the king. While the body's gender may be mistaken, the poet does recognize the figure of the king as being a body of power. This is illustrated particularly by his use of capital letters to designate *Roy*, and subsequently *Reyne*.[142]

The hermaphroditic figure provides a negative emblem that intrudes on the poet's nostalgia for the past, when the word "King" symbolized masculine strength. To reinforce the illusion that the two sexes might exist within a single body, and to substantiate his case against hermaphroditism, D'Aubigné further accentuates the ambiguities of Henry III's body by drawing from contemporary medical discourses to prove that he was a biological hermaphrodite from birth. The poet could thus claim that the representation of both illusion (the "spectacle" of the court ball) and medical knowledge were within his purview. The significance of Henry's *lubricité* (*Princes*, v. 805) is well documented in the following verses which record formative periods in his infancy and childhood.[143]

Si fut-il alaicté de poisons,
De ruzes, de conseils secrets et trahizons,
Rompu ou corrompu au trictrac des affaires,
Et eut, encore enfant, quelque part aux miseres.

(*Princes*, vv. 797–800)

Some of *Les Tragiques'* most castigating verses are based on potent symbols of condemnation (e.g., *sodomite athee*) that D'Aubigné used to distort Henry III's Catholic identity. The poet ascribes Henry's weak will and fragile body to heredity, just as he does the weak traits of his elder brother (Charles IX). In the following lines, D'Aubigné systematically describes these traits and blames them on the act of procreation, thereby impugning Catherine de Medici's and Henry II's fitness for generation.[144]

Tel fut le second fils qui n'herita du pere
Le coeur, mais les poisons et l'ame de la mere.
Le tiers par elle fut nourri et faineant,
Bien fin mais non prudent, et voulut, l'enseignant
Pour servir à son jeu, luy ordonner pour maistre
Un sodomite athee, un maquereau, un traistre.

(*Princes*, vv. 863–868)

D'Aubigné's description of Henry III as being *faineant* and "bien fin mais non prudent" supports the theory propounded in Medieval and Renaissance medical treatises (e.g., *Anatomia Magistri Nicolai Physici* and the pseudo-Galenic *De Spermate*) that hermaphroditism could be traced to conception.[145] The *De Spermate* asserts that men and women both produce seed and that all children, and therefore all hermaphrodites, were products of conflict between male and female seeds in the womb.

However, if a weak virile seed there combines with a stronger female seed, the child, though male, will be fragile in body and mind. It may even happen that from the combination of a weak male seed and a strong female seed there is born a child having both sexes.[146]

D'Aubigné's indictment of the body of the *Reyne*, Catherine de Medici, follows similar lines of corporeal deprecation. Although the poet recognized Catherine as a body of power, he focused on her savage, false and deceptive nature, depicting her as a "sauvage et carnaciere beste" (*Misères*, v. 810), by whose hand Huguenots were persecuted.

Nos cicatrices sont ton plaisir et ton jeu;
. . .
Encore ris-tu sauvage et carnaciere beste,
Aux oeuvres de tes mains, et n'as qu'un desplaisir,
Que le grand feu n'est pas si grand que ton desir!

(*Misères*, v. 803, vv. 810–812)

D'Aubigné's and Ronsard's texts are both organized around powerful corporeal lexicons. D'Aubigné offers a *physiologie* that is a testimonial to Huguenot Protestant martyrs because *Les Tragiques* reconstitutes a textual body whose inclusion in the text confirms the martyr's eternal presence. He condemns Catholics and vilifies the Catholic monarchy by denouncing its physiology, largely accomplishing this by distorting their identity. Ronsard condemned the Protestant body's physiology by accusing them of being fraudulent while attempting to rectify what he considered to be false and deceitful charges of atheism that Protestants launched at Catholics.

The opposing beliefs of these poets disclose a rivalry between two poetic discourses that generated deliberate misrepresentations of the other's physiology. Even considering the large quantity of recurring images that they used to characterize the bodies of Catholics and Protestants, the two physiologies manifest little that is positive or anatomically accurate. Instead, Ronsard and D'Aubigné both intended to demean the *physiologie* of the other religion, and in so doing often compromised the thematic stability of their poetic texts and the body of the "other."

The two poets examine the *physiologie chrestienne* through the looking glasses of their respective religions (intermingled with some physiognomy), their eyes tainted by excessive religious sentiment rather than being purified by faith, as Simon Goulart suggested.[147] They shared the same yet antithetical pedagogical goals directed at different audiences; each was determined to promote his own religion by stigmatizing the other's. Neither attempted to provide a kind or charitable view of the opposing group; neither was capable of fairly assessing and representing a *physiologie chrestienne* of the "other." They provided instead specifically vehement, retributive ones.

Throughout the poetic works examined D'Aubigné and Ronsard acted as filters in the elaboration of models of Protestant and Catholic corporeal discourse. Each celebrated his own self-image while condemning the alien or false nature of the other.

Chapter IV
Redefining Beauty: The *Oeuvres* of Louise Labé

> "Love is nothing else but a certaine coveting to enjoy beautie" (Baldassare Castiglione, *The Book of the Courtier*, 1528)

> "Women like looking at the beauty of men, as men like looking at the beauty of women" (Agnolo Firenzuola, *Dialogue on the Beauties of Women*, 1548)

Renaissance humanists described the learned woman as possessing a "manly heart" in a woman's frail body.[148] To Renaissance poetess Louise Labé (1524?-1566), scholarly women were notable because they abandoned customary female occupations in favor of literary pursuits.[149] In *Discours V* of *Le Débat de Folie et d'Amour*, a mythological prose dialogue, she asserts that literary expression is the most significant feminine artistic creation. The pen (a Renaissance symbol of the learned man)[150] and the lute replaced spinning and sewing as the means by which Labé expressed the love experience and realized her artistic potential. She exploited the link between writing and symbols of women's subjugation, e.g., the distaff and the needle, in *Discours V*, in which she wrote of women:

> Elles laissent leurs occupacions muliebres. Au lieu de filer, besongner au point, leur estude est se bien parer promener es Eglises, festes, et banquets pour avoir tousjours quelque rencontre de ce qu'elles ayment. Elles prennent la plume et le lut en main: escrivent et chantent leurs passions.[151]

Labé also formed a vision of the literate woman in the *Epitre à "A M.C.D.B.L."* (dedicated to a friend, Mademoiselle Clémence de Bourges), in which she asserted that while feminine beauty differentiated women from men, it was an inadequate distinction. She fostered an aspiration to see the feminine sex "non en beauté seulement, mais en science et vertu passer ou egaler les hommes."[152] Moreover, she declared that it was time for change; "Estant le tems venu, Madamoiselle, que les severes loix des hommes n'empeschent plus les femmes de s'apliquer aux sciences et disciplines.''[153] Labé wanted to instill in women the desire to rival men in creative enterprises by moving beyond the realm of aesthetic domestic occupations to establish a connection between women's private lives and public roles. Her renowned dedicatory epistle (which ''spells out a feminist platform for the future'' according to François Rigolot[154]) is further notable because it contains, with her use of the *nous* form, the genesis of a modern notion of female solidarity.

> Je ne puis faire autre chose que prier les vertueuses Dames d'eslever un peu leurs esprits par dessus leurs quenoilles et fuseaus, et s'employer à faire entendre au monde que si nous ne sommes faites pour commander, si ne devons nous estre desdaignees pour compagnes tant es afaires domestiques que publiques, de ceus qui gouvernent et se font obeïr.[155]

I examine in this chapter the nature of sixteenth-century views about beauty, how Louise Labé acquired a knowledge of beauty and her perception of it, and how her poetry creates an aesthetics of the body. I also describe her poetic strategy in redefining the concept of beauty, thereby forming a lover's discourse in which she appraises the masculine body and affirms that women are capable of distinguishing the qualities of beauty and creating poetry.

In addition, I elucidate Labé's reaction to the standards of Petrarchan beauty expressed in a series of poems praising her beauty by poets such as Olivier de Magny, Pontus de Tyard and Peletier du Mans. The poems appear in *Escriz de divers poëtes, à la louenge de Louize Labé Lionnoize*, which was published in the 1555 edition of her poems.[156] They construct a female subject held by her admirers to Petrarchan masculine ideals and define the feminine body as being the creation of a masculine examination of it. I analyze Labé's rejection of these commonplaces as a notion of feminine corporeal beauty. Conversely, her poems provide an interesting example of woman's writing in the way in which she articulates and manipulates questions of the structure of the masculine body.

Labé's language in *Le Débat* reveals how she interpreted the feminine and the masculine bodies as social constructs, specifically with respect to the ''perfeccion du corps ou lineament'' (*Discours V*, lines 369–370). It also reveals her efforts ''d'être charnellement vraie dans l'amour,'' and her success in creating a lover's discourse detailing ''minutieusement le processus et les jouissances ou les insatisfactions'' of love, which she considered to be the genesis of her quest for the understanding of beauty.[157] Labé expressed her opinion on what constituted corporeal beauty in her elegies and sonnets and examined ''la plaisante invencion des habits nouveaus'' at length, noting that ''tout ce qui est de beau, soit à l'acoutrement des hommes et des femmes, Amour en est l'auteur'' (*Discours V*, 383–385, of the *Débat*).

Beauty and the Primacy of Sight

In elucidating her perception of beauty, which she considered to be, above all, a quality of physical appearance, Labé subscribed to a view that evolved from a rich heritage of theoretical writings. As those works, she perceived corporeal beauty to be a property, or ingredient, of the body, which was determined by proportion; whether or not a body was beautiful was determined by whether or not it possessed the salient properties.[158] Labé's poetics focus on the beauty of the beloved and involve a sense of ''judgement of the eye''; beauty commanded her attention and pleased her eyes. Yet as will be seen, her love lyrics are grounded in scepticism about the nature and depictibility of physical beauty.[159]

To Labé, the concept of the knowability of beauty and the aesthetic perception of it were reflected in the senses of sight and hearing. She considered these senses to be the most appropriate to rational cognition, and therefore primary avenues through which she depicted beauty in her poetry. Beauty consisted in qualities shared in common by objects appealing to both of these senses.[160] Labé's considered sight to be the most exalted sense; its presence is evident throughout her work. One must consider it to understand her perception of the body's visual beauty because her clearest knowledge of it derives from that sense. She frequently stresses the subjective aspect of visual contemplation and the role of pleasure in experiencing beauty.

> O dous regars, o yeus pleins de beauté
> Petis jardins, pleins de fleurs amoureuses
> Où sont d'Amour les flesches dangereuses,
> Tant à vous voir mon oeil s'est arresté!
> . . .
> Donques, mes yeus, tant de plaisir avez,
> Tant de bons tours par ses yeus recevez:
>
> (Sonnet 11, vv. 1–4, 9–10)

Often her poems articulate the corporeal absence of the beloved and command the beloved's presence through the visual element of the stellar eye of ''Clere Venus, qui erres par les Cieus'' (S. 5, v. 1).

> Mon oeil veillant s'atendira bien mieus,
> Et plus de pleurs te voyant getera.
> Mieux mon lit mol de larmes baignera,
> De ses travaus voyant témoins tes yeus.
>
> (Sonnet 5, vv. 5–8)

Labé stresses the senses in the ultimate portrayal of the concrete phenomena of beauty. However, rather than always relying on visual experience to communicate corporeal beauty and to depict the masculine body, she also relies heavily on imagination, to form a spiritual vision of an absent corporeal body that will appear later.

Sonnet 20 should be examined with these factors in mind. The poem contains a striking example of the theory popularized by Pléiade poets that the imagination can envision events and persons not previously experienced. The poetess creates a fantasy based upon a fortune teller's prognostication which permitted her to control events at the first meeting with a predestined lover. The first quatrain fashions a mental image of the masculine body characterized as the object of a woman's scrutiny (''celui dont la figure / Me fut descrite''). The quatrain concludes with allusions to visual perception although the lover does not appear physically. Labé has used this ability to observe absent corporeal things to stress the superiority of the spiritual vision over the corporeal sense of vision.

Predit me fut, que devoit fermement
Un jour aymer celui dont la figure
Me fut descrite: et sans autre peinture
Le reconnu quand vy premierement:

(Sonnet 20, vv. 1–4)

In discerning beauty, Labé preferred to employ the power of her own feminine gaze (''Tant emploiray de mes yeus le pouvoir'' S. 6 v. 12). She queries how to represent the image of the utopian beloved in her well-known ''portrait'' sonnet 21, in which she attempts to evoke the male's presence by manipulating the architectural components of the body into a collage of the desired object. This takes the form of a descriptive catalogue. In calling attention to the architecture of the body, Labé reflects the aesthetic preoccupations of the female literary culture. And as Ann Rosalind Jones notes, she also affirms the lack of a desiderata for describing the masculine body.[161]

Labé concurred with the dominant sixteenth-century art theory by identifying beauty in Sonnet 21 with a sense of proportion that gave pleasure. She regarded corporeal beauty to be as much a matter of quantity (*Quelle grandeur?*, *Quelle grosseur?*) as quality *quel poil?*, *quelle couleur . . . des yeus?*). Ultimately, she developed what she believed to be a sense of perfection through the fundamental aesthetic qualities of eye color, complexion, and shades of beard, head of hair, or both.

Quelle grandeur rend l'homme venerable?
Quelle grosseur? quel poil? quelle couleur?
Qui est des yeus le plus emmieleur?

(Sonnet 21, vv. 1–3)

Conversely, in contemplating the sensuous form, Labé also identified grace as a quality of beauty. This was revealed particularly through a sense of vocal and aural harmony of the *lut* and the *chant* performed together to permit the perception of the masculine physical being. In the following quatrain, the poetess proclaims the role of poetry and the status of the poet as one that will reveal the true character of the man's voice.

Quel chant est plus à l'homme convenable?
Qui plus penetre en chantant sa douleur?
Qui un dous lut fait encore meilleur?
Quel nature est le plus amiable?

(Sonnet 21, vv. 5–8)

In the same context, she asserted in an earlier sonnet that her role as poetic *persona* qualified her to sing the *graces* of the lover in an attempt to comprehend and depict him.

Tant que ma main pourra les cordes tendre
Du mignart Lut, pour tes graces chanter:
Tant que l'esprit se voudra contenter
De ne vouloir rien fors que toy comprendre:
Je ne souhaitte encore point mourir.
. . .

(Sonnet 14, vv. 5–9)

Labé's poems articulate the corporeal absence of the beloved and serve as a substitute, forming a corporeal discourse that is the *lierre* that binds lovers' bodies together in a treatise of love that is, as Michel de Certeau observes, a story articulated by bodies, just as all love stories are.[162]

Oh si j'estois en ce beau sein ravie
De celui là pour lequel vois mourant:
. . .
Si de mes bras le tenant acollé,
Comme du Lierre est l'arbre encercelé,
. . .

(Sonnet 13, vv. 1–2, 9–10)

The central lesson of "portrait" sonnet 21 is the fact that one governed by the power of love cannot logically measure masculine beauty. Labé uses the term *jugement* to connote sensible knowledge, as if its meaning were already known. The term, which retains its common meaning of evaluation or discrimination, becomes the means by which she avows her artistic inadequacy, or at least tries to deal with the inexpressibility topos in the experience of beauty and love.[163] In her search for beauty, Labé casts doubt on the possibility of finding even the perimeters of beauty. The mythological figure of Love, *Amour* clouds her judgment, making it impossible for her to measure adequately the qualities of masculine beauty.

Je ne voudrois le dire assurément
Ayant Amour forcé mon jugement:
Mais je say bien et de tant je m'assure,
Que tout le beau que l'on pourroit choisir,
Et que tout l'art que ayde la Nature,
Ne me sauroient acroitre mon desir.

(Sonnet 21, vv. 9–14)

Idealized Corporeal Beauty: Petrarchan Excesses

Most of Labé's sonnets deal to some extent with beauty as a male attribute; indeed, she characterizes the masculine body more fully than the feminine, yet she does not neglect female beauty. She suggests that while beauty was largely considered to be a woman's attribute by contemporary male poets, corporeal beauty was essentially for males to admire, whether it be in females or males. To write as a woman, Labé had to refocus this consideration of beauty. One of her poetic strategies was to note that male poets went to extremes in describing female beauty lavishing highly stereotyped epithets on women in attempting to delineate their attributes. In analyzing beauty, she refers specifically to poems that submit her to the masculine ideal of Petrarchan praise, and she refuses to endorse the power of masculine poetic discourse although it informs the Renaissance model of womanly beauty.[164] Lawrence Kritzman categorizes the Petrarchan system of portraying the female body as one "through which male writers fetishize the female body and dismember it through their scriptural practices."[165] Labé used the representation of her own beauty by contemporary poets as a poetic strategy to study critically this aspect of a male poet's descriptions of the idealized corporeal attributes of his beloved.

In *Elégie II* Labé indicates what differentiates her from a possible rival. She postulates a different woman, perhaps a more natural one, with her real charms concealed behind the patriarchial textual facade. Yet she apparently doubts the male poets' appreciation of her own beauty; this is confirmed by expressions such as "plusieurs gens. . . / M'ont fait à tort, . . . estre estimee." This doubt resurfaces in her statement "tu me l'as fait croire," in which she acknowledges that the poet, in this case Olivier de Magny, had led her to believe that numerous poets in Italy had praised her.

Si say je bien que t'amie nouvelle
A peine aura le renom d'estre telle,
Soit en beauté, vertu, grace et faconde,

Comme plusieurs gens savans par le monde
M'ont fait à tort, ce croy je, estre estimee.
Mais qui pourra garder la renommee?
Non seulement en France suis flatee,
Et beaucoup plus, que ne veus, exaltee.
. . .
Le beau païs auquel or'te promeines,
Ont entendu (tu me l'as fait croire)
Que gens d'esprit me donnent quelque gloire.
(*Elégie II*, vv. 55–62, 66–68)[166]

Elsewhere, Labé continues to base her analysis of the lexical excesses of male poets on a more worldly aspect of feminine beauty depicted in the Petrarchan lexicon: "le petit pie." She notes in her *Discours V*, 379–381: "le plus souvent l'amoureuse curiosité des hommes fait rechercher la beauté jusques au bout des piez."[167] Pontus de Tyard searches for the origins of Labé's divine beauty in a sonnet in *Escriz* entitled "En contemplacion de dame Louise Labé." He uses an appeal that suggests a pattern of stolen beauty, perhaps from the gods: "De quel lys est, mais de quelle Deesse / Cette beauté, qui les autres destrousse?"[168] De Magny praises Labé's beauty in another sonnet in the same collection, in which he uses a lexicon that exploits examples of perfection found typically in traditional Petrarchan poems. He fuses them with references to standard mythological parallels, again suggesting beauty acquired from the gods.[169]

Où print l'enfant Amour le fin or qui dora
En mille crespillons ta teste blondissante?
. . .
Et les raiz de cet oeil qui doucement m'enchante,
En quel lieu les prit-il quand il t'en decora?
. . .
Prit-il d'Herme, de Cypre et du lict de l'aurore,
Des rayons du soleil et des Graces encore, . . .?
(*Les Soupirs*, S. 32 vv. 1–2, 7–8, 12–13)

Labé again denotes her awareness of the excesses of Petrarchan love poetry in Sonnet 23, in which she tries to extricate herself from de Magny's poetic image of her, and therefore from the Petrarchan poetic convention of describing the "fragmented" beauty of a passive beloved female.

Las! que me sert, que si parfaitement
Louas jadis et ma tresse doree,
Et de mes yeus la beauté comparee
A deus Soleils, dont Amour finement
. . .
Tira les trets causez de ton tourment?

Où estes vous, pleurs de peu de duree?
Et Mort par qui devoit estre honoree
Ta ferme amour et iteré serment?

(Sonnet 23, vv. 1–4, 5–8)

While attacking Petrarchan excesses, Labé also assails the lover's indifference and insincerity. She rejects the male poet's praise and, to demonstrate her unwillingness to yield to the power of his examination, she refuses to be transformed into an object of contemplation. Instead, by stating ''Las! que me sert,'' she deprives the male poet (de Magny) of his power, thus demonstrating that she considers Petrarchan amorous conquest to be an empty cliché.

Verbal Disfigurations of Feminine Beauty

In *Elégie I*, Labé moves from a discussion of love to an analysis of beauty in which she develops the concept of beauty as a negative and retributive power. A *carpe florem* that ends the elegy dramatically represents the artistic struggle to recover lost beauty and youth. This is illustrated in the lamentations of an old woman who, ''having scorned love in her youth, now suffers the pangs of passion. She tries frantically to restore the beauty with which she once attracted potential lovers,'' yet the lover she once spurned now rejects her.[170] The relationship between beauty and betrayal in this elegy is a close one, and provided Labé with a language to describe and analyze the physical attributes of beauty. As such, the gift of beauty is replaced because of aging by an illusion of beauty in Labé's elegy. A kind of personal involvement appears in her allusion to a distinction between youth and old age, and reappears later in a juxtaposition of beauty and ugliness as she narrates the experiences of a woman who ''essayoit se faire venir belle'' (v. 100).

Telle j'ai vu qui avoit en jeunesse
Blamé Amour: après en sa vieillesse
Bruler d'ardeur, et pleindre tendrement
L'âpre rigueur de son tardif tourment.

(*Elégie I*, vv. 95–98)

Elégie I represents a change of focus in Labé's depiction of beauty. She esteems the aesthetic, yet shuns artificial beauty, and thus addresses the Renaissance period condemnation of embellishing the body with artificial products. In the sonnets discussed earlier, she focuses on well-formed, natural beauty, which is generally a physical beauty belonging to youth, and presents a definite ideal of beauty in which she lauds the symmetry of the body's members, comparing them to harmonic tones in a melody. Labé goes far beyond her representation of the body in the sonnets by portraying the old woman in a series of lexical disfigurations in which she describes the transformations of the body's surfaces and contours through the process of aging, and the old woman's futile attempts to conceal those changes and restore youthful beauty by means of *fard*, *eau continuelle*, and *quelque perruque*. Labé also depicts her former lover's spurning as punishment for her youthful arrogance.

Alors de fard et eau continuelle
Elle essayoit se faire venir belle,
Voulant chasser le ridé labourage,
Que l'aage avoit gravé sur son visage.
Sur son chef gris elle avoit empruntee
Quelque perruque, et assez mal antee:
Et plus estoit à son gré bien fardee,
De son ami moins estoit regardee:
Lequel ailleurs fuiant n'en tenoit conte,
Tant lui sembloit laide, et avoit grand'honte
D'estre aymé d'elle. Ainsi la pauvre vieille
Recevoit bien pareille pour pareille.

(*Elégie*, I vv. 99–110)

Contemplation of the love object and the struggle to define corporeal beauty were common themes in Renaissance love poetry. As we have seen, poets often promoted the notion inherited from the Petrarchan tradition that feminine corporeal beauty was best described by ennumerating bodily parts, and therefore incorporated all the conventional aspects of beauty in their meticulously written poetry. Conversely, we have seen how Labé recognized the limitations of mere recitation and how she struggled with the problem of rendering a more accurate portrayal of the complete essence of masculine corporeal beauty. Although she approached a poetic evocation of the masculine body in her choice of a visual theme, she disappoints the reader by failing to express adequately the lover's beauty, or to describe precisely his body. She relies instead on the inexpressibility topos, much the same as we have seen in Petrarchan poetry. However, a far different representation of the feminine body appears in Labé's poetry. Although she found her inspiration for the sense of beauty in the work of sixteenth-century male poets, she sought to redefine the composition of feminine corporeal loveliness by adequately distinguishing woman not by her bodily beauties alone, but as a worthy intellectual rival of man. identity of his subjects for more clarity.

Conclusion: Renaissance Representation

The human body, perhaps the most obvious fact of human existence, is a subject about which French Renaissance poets had a great deal to say. As illustrated in this study, the sixteenth century nurtured an important poetic discourse of the body. By tracing the language of the body in each poetic text chosen for this study, the major concerns of sixteenth century poets have emerged. These poems reveal that interest in the body was not restricted to scientific poetry, but overlapped other genres, e.g., the satirical, moral and lyrical, in which the essence of the human body is carefully examined.

Religious beliefs and practices in Creation poetry provide the starting point for molding models of the body. However, Creation poets drew on both biblical and medical traditions to reassemble the story of Creation into a wider and more pervasive theory of man the microcosm that represented him both as a medical model, and as a social system. This study illustrates that the poetic debate over the nature and importance of the body in sixteenth century society reflected both reorganization of medical theories relating to the science of anatomy, and the growing awareness of the changing symbolic significance of the body in relation to that scientific development. This urge to analyze, define, and classify the structure of the body in poetic discourse was also a response to the concern for expanding the resources of the French language, and for drawing on the vast knowledge contained in ancient Greek and Latin literary sources.

Above all, one finds that the narration of Genesis in Creation poems is a strong connecting link between them. These poetic discourses reveal, however, that each poet's perception of the body was based on the individual voice of a poet embarked on a unique spiritual adventure. While many of these poems are impossibly extravagant, especially those by Du Bartas, the world of the poem provided no means to capture fully the intricacy of the body's structure. Du Bartas and D'Aubigné, for whom ''represanter'' meant ''peindre par le discours,'' [171] both sought to create splendid poetry to represent the body of man, yet neither poet was able to realize fully his aspiration to describe the body with the finesse found in Greek and Latin medical works. They were never fully satisfied with their poetic accomplishments. Consequently, frustration is mirrored in their verses. Legendary figures such as Aesculapius, Galen, and Herophilus, men of magnificent medical achievements, lurk in the background of the structure of their poems.

The representation of the body in the poems of François Béroalde De Verville and Joseph Du Chesne reflects changes in moral and societal values during the Renaissance. They viewed the human body as an historical and cultural reality to be constantly reinterpreted. As such they provided extremely interesting social documents, yet the inadequacy of poetry as a medium for ''truth'' is apparent in their works. While sixteenth century scientific poets proposed to incorporate scientific methods into their compositions, we observe that the texts repeatedly question the validity and the probability of accomplishing this in any exhaustive manner. In poetic discourse the cold logic required to examine scientifically the body's anatomy is often transformed into a distinctively artistic reproduction of the body in verse. This process often becomes an imaginary journey manipulated by the poet's ''docte main.''

In practice, Du Bartas, D'Aubigné, Béroalde De Verville, Du Chesne and others idealized the bodies about which they wrote. Their panegyric representations surpassed the reality found in anatomical texts. This does not mean that they failed to represent the body, or that prose provided the only means to the ''truth.'' Rather, the goal of poetry and the role of the poet differed from that found in prose. Marcel Thiry's examination of the role of the poet facilitates the understanding of the difference between poetry and prose. He argues that

> Le poète modifie, c'est sa fonction. Nous savons, et cette étymologie n'est que trop souvent rappelée, que le poète est celui qui fait. Mais le prosateur aussi invente et fabrique; le don du poète est de changer la nature de ce qu'il touche. La vue des choses ni les lois de la société ne sont plus les mêmes après que l'aventure poétique les a rencontrées et traversées.[172]

Du Bellay's *Regrets* confirm the importance that he attached to Greek and Latin medical works in examining the poet's status in society. He incorporated medicine and humoral psychology in the *Regrets* in order to delineate and validate the textual body of the poetic *persona*, and argued in *La Deffence et illustration de la langue françoyse* that ''if poets were to leave pictures of nature that matched the excellence of those presented in the ancient world, they would need to rebuild the entire fabric of poetry.''[173] Du Bellay set out to reconstruct poetry, which he considered to be an art ''capable of expressing the living energy of nature.''[174]

Ronsard is perhaps the only poet to implement fully the reforms suggested by Du Bellay. He states in his *Abbrégé poétique* that poetry, just as the living body, must consist of ''belles inventions, descriptions, comparaisons, qui font les ners & la vie du livre'' that the poet could use as key concepts in expressing poetically the sense of mystery surrounding the human body.

Similarly, Ronsard and D'Aubigné's challenge to one another in their analysis of the ''physiologie chrestienne,'' in which each focuses on the human body as a locus for representing social and religious critique reveals a poetic discourse which generated deliberate misrepresentations of both the Protestant and the Catholic bodies.

The analysis of Labé's brief corpus of lyric poems provides a glimpse of the female poet's contemplation of the male body. Examining two meanings of Renaissance ''aesthetics,'' Labé relates imagination to a specific type of visual experience of the characteristics of the masculine body, and expresses the need to redefine feminine beauty. She bases that redefinition on what contemporary poets said about beautiful women.

Considering the ultimate purpose of this study, which is to explain how Renaissance poets represented the body in their work, it is perhaps fitting to examine the role of the poet and the nature of poetry itself. A remark by Leonardo da Vinci in comparing poetry unfavorably to painting is apt: ''Whereas painting is born in the light of nature, poetry is born in the *occhio tenebroso* of the imagination.''[175] More recently, the poet has been defined as being one who ''reveals the deepest feelings of his soul with sincerity and authenticity and who discovers, then transmits to the reader, secrets of the universe.''[176]

While the sixteenth-century poet perhaps did not consider sincerity or authenticity to be requisite to their art, they were nonetheless aware that one of their principal roles was to reveal the structure of the body and other secrets of the universe. They were also aware of the nature and the limitations of the poetic enterprise, and thus that fully illuminating the nature of the body was impossible. The sixteenth-century alliance of anatomy and poetry produced a poet betwixt two worlds, reality and a painted canvas, who attempted to represent both in the mind of the observer. However, if the empirical methods of sixteenth-century scientific thought were intended to reveal the ''truth'' about the structure of the human body, contemporary poetry illustrates that the body became an idealistic expression of the poet's observations. Scientific consciousness was often blurred deliberately. The sixteenth-century poet fused prose with poetry to create a new poetry that incorporated what some twentieth century critics consider to be nonpoetic values, e.g., the emotive, the moral, and the epistemological.

In concluding, it is apparent that the sixteenth-century poet was a craftsman, a satirist, and a moralist who was useful to society and worked in harmony with it. But it should be remembered that Renaissance poets were intimately involved in all aspects of the quest to know man. They sought to transform old forms and patterns and to create new ones; above all they hoped to advance the causes of poetry and the French language. All sixteenth-century Creation poets and poets of the human body had two things in common: a desire to express in poetic form what many esteemed could not be said as gracefully or as eloquently in prose, and a belief in their own crucial, unique importance as poets to transmit knowledge.

> Le poète est celui qui sait, celui qui a cheminé tout au long d'une voie mystérieuse pour arriver au Temple et en franchir le seuil sacré, avant de contempler la Réalité face à face, de saisir ''les splendeurs situées derrière le tombeau.'' [177]

Notes

1. Lengthy accounts and definitions of the woman's body are found in Renaissance writings. Significantly, many of them concern matters of sex differences, and distinguish woman by a different bodily makeup than man. They often present synthetic views of her that are drawn from a stock of commonplaces derived from ancient traditions, particularly Aristotelian, of imagining gender differences. See the excellent study by Ian Maclean, *The Renaissance Notion of Woman*, Cambridge, Cambridge University Press, 1980, and my study of gender, below.

2. Pierre de La Primaudaye, *Académie françoise* (1581) (Slatkine Reprints, Genève, 1972), "Du corps & de l'Ame," Ch.II, 6.

3. Numerous theologians challenged this view of the female body during the Renaissance. In particular, Martin Luther, in his commentaries on Genesis I:27, disavows that woman is an imperfect version of the male, and asserts that those who propound such a view "are themselves monsters and the sons of monsters." See Maclean, 9.

4. Charles Estienne, *La dissection des parties du corps divisee en trois livres*, Paris, Simon de Colines, 1546. Ch.4.2.

5. However, the frontispiece of the monumental work of Andreas Vesalius, *The Epitome*, published in 1543, depicts the anatomist beside the anatomized body of a woman. See R.L. Lind, *The Epitome of Andreas Vesalius*, Cambridge, Mass., The M.I.T. Press, 1949.

6. Pierre de Ronsard, *Abbregé de l'art poëtique françois* (1565) (Slatkine Reprints, Genève, 1972), 5.

7. *Fragments for a History of the Human Body*. Eds. Michel Feher with Ramona Naddaff and Nadia Tazi. Zone, New York, 1989, Part 3., p. 454.

8. *Fragments*, 465. Paracelsus (1490–1541), celebrated Swiss physician, chemist, and natural philosopher.

9. The microcosm-macrocosm analogy was associated with Pythagoras (6th c. B.C.), who formulated the first cosmology. Pythagorean cosmology flourished throughout the Medieval period into the Renaissance. It withstood periodic

challenges, and although weakened was not repudiated until the scientific revolution. It was through Plato's writings, especially the *Timaeus*, the basic text for cosmology, that the Pythagorean doctrine influenced the Renaissance. See S.K. Heninger, *Touches of Sweet Harmony, Pythagorean Cosmology and Renaissance Poetics*, San Marino, California, The Huntington Library, 1979.

10. This was the traditional Medieval portrait of man as microcosm propounded in the twelfth century by Alain de Lille and illustrated in the *Elucidarium* of Honoré d'Autun. The *Elucidarium* contains one of the early European depictions of man as a microcosmic figure, "[O]n y voit, encadré dans un rectangle qui porte aux quatre coins les symboles des éléments, un homme se dresser debout, nu et gracile, sur une plante stylisée; une auréole, rappelant la sphère céleste, entoure sa tête aux longues cheveux; d'étroits phylactères où sont inscrits le nom des cinq planètes et des luminaires jaillissent de ses yeux, de ses narines, de ses oreilles, de sa bouche; le mot air orne sa poitrine, le mot mer s'imprime sur son ventre, le mot terre désigne ses pieds; quatre banderoles portant l'explication élémentaire des cinq sens rejoignent les monogrammes des quatres éléments." in Albert-Marie Schmidt, *La Poésie scientifique en France au seizième siècle*, Lausanne, Editions Rencontre, 1970, 140.

11. Schmidt, 140–41.

12. *Michel de Montaigne Essais*, Texte établi et annoté par Albert Thibaudet, Bibliothèque de la Pléiade, Paris, 1940, II, xvii, 625.

13. Donald M. Frame, *Montaigne's Discovery of Man*, New York, Columbia University Press, 1955, 81.

14. Frame, 1955, 81.

15. Essais, II, xii, 521.

16. Essais, II, xii, 522.

17. Schmidt, 141.

18. This is a celebrated maxim taken from the *Emerald Table*, an ancient hermetic text ascribed to Hermes that contained the basic laws of alchemy. See Grillot de Givry, *Witchcraft, Magic and Alchemy*, trans. J. Courtenay Locke ([New York:] Frederick Publications, 1954), 240.

19. Verdun-L. Saulnier, *Maurice Scève*, (Genève, Slatkine Reprints, 1981), vol. I, 407.

20. The zodiacal signs and the parts of the anatomy to which they correspond are as follows: The Ram (Aries)—the head, The Bull—(Taurus) the neck, The Twins (Gemini)—the arms, The Lion (Leo)—the shoulders, The Crab (Cancer)—the breast, The Maiden (Virgo)—the entrails, The Scales (Libra)—the buttocks, The Scorpion (Scorpio)—the genitals, The Centaur (Sagitarius)—the thighs, The Goat (Capricornus)—the knees, The Water Bearer (Aquarius)—the lower legs, The Fish (Pisces)—the feet. "It was thus possible to envision the zodiac as a great man lying in a circle with his head in Aries and his feet at Pisces. And because

of the astrological associations of planets with the zodiacal signs, the correlation of the heavens with man was both anatomical and psychological.'' George Boas, in *Dictionary of the History of Ideas*, ed. Philip P. Wiener, New York, Charles Scribner's Sons, c. 1973, Vol. III, 128.

21. Maurice Scève, *Oeuvres complètes,* texte établi et annoté par Pascal Quignard, Mercure de France, Paris, 1974, 247, Bk. I, vv. 121–23, 131,137.

22. The superiority of man over woman, particularly in matters pertaining to the deduction of sexual differences, is expounded in many Renaissance texts. This belief derives to a certain extent from both Ancient and Medieval thought, e.g., Aristotle and St Thomas Aquinas. Both present the notion of woman as being inferior, or as an imperfect male. Aristotle, in a well-known passage of the *De generatione animalium* (II.3 [838a 27]), bases his description of the female as an incomplete male upon a series of paired dualities such as male/female, ''active/passive, form/matter, act/potency, perfection/imperfection, completion/ incompletion, possession/deprivation.'' Ian Maclean (*The Renaissance Notion of Woman*, 8).

    Aquinas incorporates Aristotle's view, and provides his own understanding of the position of women as one not of ''. . . something manqué, but is according to the plan of nature ['*intentio naturae*'], and is directed towards the work of procreation.'' (Maclean, p 9). It is this conception of woman as an imperfect male that met with considerable hostility from theologians such as Martin Luther. He denounced the unfavorable figurative associations found in Aristotle and Aquinas despite the fact that this view was consistent with his own belief in woman's inferiority to man.

    In his commentary on Genesis (I: 27), Luther states:

    > '' . . . it is evident therefore that woman is a different animal to man, not only having different members, but also being far weaker in intellect [ingenium]. But although Eve was a most noble creation, like Adam, as regards the image of God, that is, in justice, wisdom and salvation, she was none the less a woman . . . . so also woman, although the most beautiful handiwork of God, does not equal the dignity and glory of the male.'' Maclean, pp 9–10.

23. Guillaume de Saluste Du Bartas, *La Sepmaine*, édition établie, présentée et annotée par Yvonne Bellenger, Librairie Nizet, Paris, 1981. I have used Bellenger's edition for all citations of Du Bartas' poem, except where indicated.

24. Du Bartas' idea of the *Quinta Essentia* may have been inspired by the doctrine of the ''Predestined Element'' found in passages from Aristotle's *De Generatione et Corruptione* II, 3 and 4. These deal with a cycle of transformations. In ''each object one of the elements acquires a power superior to that of the others—and it is this element which forms the kernel of the object. It embodies all its specific power and virtues and thereby marks the essential difference of one object from another.'' See Walter Pagel, *Paracelsus, An Introduction to Philosophical Medicine in the Era of the Renaissance*, 2nd, revised edition, Karger, Basel, 1982, 83. A similar idea was developed by Paracelsus, for whom the ''fifth essences'' were intrinsic virtues which were the very spirit of life, but were without shape or form, ''not outwardly visible, . . . not in the shape of bodies.'' Pagel, 56.

25. Simon Goulart observes that Du Bartas ''set downe the grossest traces of this admirable table, for the pleasure and content of those, who are least experienced in these things.'' *A learned summarie upon the famous poeme of William of Salust, lord of Bartas: wherein are discovered all the excellent secrets in metaphysicall, physicall, morall, and historicall knowledge . . . /translated out of . . .* London: Printed for R.M., 1636, 268.

26. Guillaume de la Perrière, *Le Théâtre des Bons Engins auquel sont contenuz cent Emblemes moraulx* (1539), Scholars' Facsimiles & Reprints, Gainsville, Florida, 1964, 80–81.

27. ''Comme ainsi soit que nous feussions espars, comme brebis esgarées par le laberynthe de ce monde: il nous a recueillis pour nous assembler avec soy.'' Jean Calvin, *Institutes de la Religion Chrétienne*. XVII, 785, cited in Edmond Huguet, Dictionnaire de la Langue française du seizième siècle, Didier, Paris, 1950, ''labyrinth,'' vol. 4, 748.

   Huston Diehl suggests that Protestant theology shaped the image of the labyrinth during the Renaissance. The image is present in Calvin's *Institutes*, and was undoubtedly known to Protestant poets. See Huston Diehl, ''Into the maze of the self: the Protestant transformation of the image of the labyrinth,'' in *The Journal of Medieval and Renaissance Studies*, Vol. 16, No. 2, Fall 1986, 297–8.

28. Du Bartas also describes the ears, drawing largely from Aristotelian thought, as ''Portieres de l'esprit, escoutes de nos corps / Vrais juges des accents, huissieres des thresors'' (vv. 599–600).

29. The *sacquebute*, or *saquebute*, is a wind instrument like the trombone used in the Middle Ages. See Paul Robert, *Dictionnaire Alphabétique & Analogique de la Langue Française*, Paris, 1978, 1748.

30. Diehl contends that Protestantism ''alters man's relation to the objective, visible world, encouraging believers to look inward.'' See his ''Into the maze of the self,'' n. 27.

31. *La Création* was written in Geneva near the end of the poet's life. For further background on this poem see Keith Cameron, *Agrippa D'Aubigné*, Twayne Publishers, Boston, 1977, 142–143, and Théodore Agrippa d'Aubigné, *Oeuvres complètes*, éds. Réaume & De Caussade, Alphonse Lemerre, Paris, 1874, T. III., 327–417.

32. See Cameron, *Agrippa D'Aubigné*, 142–43.

33. The last five *Chants* treat man, his body and soul; xi-xiii pertain to the body, while xiv and xv detail the nature and actions of the soul.

34. Lyndy Abraham, *Marvell and Alchemy*, Aldershot, Hants, England, Scolar Press, 1991, 91.

35. Béroalde strongly echoes Paracelsian views that man is a microcosm composed of four elements. He also shared many of Paracelsus' alchemical beliefs. For a discussion of Paracelsus see George Perrigo Conger, *Theories of Macrocosms and Microcosms in the History of Philosophy*. New York, Russell & Russell, reissued,

1967, 55–60, and Walter Pagel, *Paracelsus, An Introduction to Philosophical Medicine in the Era of the Renaissance*. Basel, Karger, 1982.

36. *Les Cognoissances*, f. 11v.

37. Stephen Bamforth, "Béroalde de Verville and the question of scientific poetry," *Renaissance and Modern Studies*, vol. xxiii, 1979, 125.

38. *Les Cognoissances*, dedicatory pieces.

39. Bamforth notes: "The alchemist sees himself in some sense at least as continuing God's work in creation," in "Béroalde de Verville . . . ," 110.

40. The Hermetic vessel contains three primordial forces (sulphur, quicksilver and salt; spirit; soul and body). Together they form the alchemical *Tria prima* and constitute the nature of the corporeal world and man. *Le transport aux cieux* is mercury, or quicksilver, which because of its white color symbolizes the moon, and the feminine element. Quicksilver also represents the *primus agens* that alchemists considered to be a manifestation of the first matter. Sulphur, because of its coloring power, represents the essence of gold, the sun, and the masculine element. Salpetre, the salt, represents the static or neutral element, and the body of man. Titus Burckhardt notes: "Transposed to man, salt is not simply the body in its outward form, it is its psychic form, and as such has a twofold aspect." *Alchemy: Science of the Cosmos, Science of the Soul*, trans. William Stoddart, Penguin Books, Baltimore, 1972, 147, 165–66.

41. The term *vaine* signified "emptie, void, without purpose," *terre vaine* was "A wast ground; or a ground which hath neither feed in, nor fruit upon, it." Cotgrave.

42. Joseph du Chesne, sieur de la Violette, *L'anatomie du petit monde, avec quelques sonnets des vices d'icelui*, s.l., 1584. B. Arsenal: 4° B.L. 3168.

43. Joseph Du Chesne, *L'Anatomie*, pièces limnaires, n. pag.

44. Cotgrave defines *Dameret* as, "an effeminate fondling, or fond carpet knight; one that spends his whole time in the intertaining, or courting, of women."

45. *The Epitome of Andreas Vesalius*, trans. L.R. Lind, Cambridge, Mass., The M.I.T. Press, 1949, xvii. *The Epitome*, a descriptive anatomy, summarized material contained in the seven books of the *Fabrica*, and is thought to have been intended for use as an aid to medical students. See Lind, 9.

46. Vesalius, "Dedicatory Letter to Philip II", *Epitome*, xxxiv.

47. Ambroise Paré, "Au Lecteur", *Oeuvres complètes*, ed. by J.-F. Malgaigne, (Slatkine Reprints, Genève, 1970), Tome I, 15.

48. Paré, "Au Lecteur," 15.

49. Paré, *Introduction à la Chirurgie*, Ch. IV., 33.

50. A. Wear notes that the head-to-toe order, known as the *practica*, was found in Galen and in other anatomical works throughout the sixteenth century and

remained standard practice until the appearance of Theophile Bonet's *Mercurius Compilatitius* (1682), which substituted an alphabetical listing of diseases. See A. Wear, ''Explorations in Renaissance Writings,'' *The Medical Renaissance of the Sixteenth-Century*, eds., A. Wear, R.K. French and I.M. Lonie, Cambridge, Cambridge University Press, 1985, 126–7.

51. Paré, *Oeuvres Complètes*, Tome, I, ''Premier Livre, Traitant de l'anatomie de tout le corps humain,'' Ch. I ''Division du corps humain,'' 108.

52. However, recent attention has been given to Du Bartas' scientific poetry. See James Dauphiné, *Guillaume de Saluste Du Bartas poète scientifique*, Paris, Société D'Edition ''Les Belles Lettres,'' 1983, and *Du Bartas poète encyclopédique du XVIe siècle*, Colloque international, faculté des lettres et sciences humaines de Pau et des pays de l'Adour 7, 8 et 9 mars 1986, ed. James Dauphiné, Lyon, La Manufacture, 1988.

53. The *Epitome* contains the following: Book I Bones and Cartilage, II Muscles and Ligaments, III Abdominal Viscera, IV Thoracic Viscera and Vascular System, V The Brain and the Nervous System, and VI Organs of Reproduction. See Lind, xxiv.

54. To compare more fully D'Aubigné's and Vesalius' interpretations, see Lind, 69–71.

55. Paré, *Oeuvres Complètes*, Tome I, ''Le Troisième Livre de L'Anatomie contenant les parties animales situées en la teste,'' Ch. I, ''Description generale de la teste,'' 210.

56. Paré, 212 & 214.

57. Cotgrave defines *amasseur* as ''A piler, heaper, gatherer; a taker up of, or stooper for, things.''

58. However, the use of the head-to-toe structure to organize his anatomy and the thoroughness of his examination strongly suggest that D'Aubigné intended this poem to be a teaching piece, presumably for his son Nathan, as others have suggested.

59. Marie-Christine Pouchelle has studied the continuity of the use of offices to designate different functions of the body, as well as its socio-religious connotations. See *Corps et Chirurgie à l'Apogée du Moyen-Age*, Paris, Flammarion, 1983, 194–196.

60. The social body metaphor, borrowed from Aristotelian thought, was already a well-established feature of Medieval medicine that continued to be used in the Renaissance. See Pouchelle, 194–6.

61. D'Aubigné, *Oeuvres*, V. III, 240–43.

62. Urban Tigner Holmes, Jr., *The Works of Guillaume de Salluste Sieur Du Bartas: A Critical Edition with Introduction, Commentary, and Variants*, 3 Vols., Chapel Hill, The University of North Carolina Press, 1935, I, 220.

63. On the affinities of art and poetry see Rensselaer W. Lee, "Ut pictura poesis: The Humanistic Theory of Painting", *Art Bulletin* 22 (1940): 197–269 (reprint, New York, 1967); E.H. Gombrich, *Symbolic Images: Studies in the Art of the Renaissance* (London, 1972). See also Margaret M. McGowan, *Ideal Forms in the Age of Ronsard* (University of California Press, Berkeley, 1985). An additional reference to the intimate links between the "sister arts" may be found in Blaise de Vigenère's, *Les Images des deux Philostrates grecs* (Paris, 1578) published several years before Du Bartas' *Brief Advertissement.* Blaise de Vigenère wrote: "La poesie est une peinture parlante, / et la peinture une poesie muette." Cited in McGowan, 51. See also Simonides' statement that, "Painting is a dumme Poesie, and a Poesie is a speaking painting." Cited in Norman K. Farmer, Jr., *Poets and the Visual Arts in Renaissance England*, Austin, University of Texas Press, 1984, ix.

64. Franc Ducros, "Entre l'oeil et la main: du défaut à l'exces," in *La Représentation du corps dans la culture italienne*, Actes du Colloque de 1982, Centre d'Etudes Italiennes d'Aix-en Provence, Université de Provence, 1983, 88.

65. Guillaume de Saluste du Bartas, *La Sepmaine* (Texte de 1581), Ed. par Yvonne Bellenger, Paris, Nizet, 1981, 279.

66. The comparison *ut pictura poesis* is Bellenger's, 296.

67. This *épître* was dedicated to Jean De Brosses who, according to Jacques Pineaux, "appartenait à une famille noble de la Bresse. Il possédait des biens près de Genève, et occupait une place ce conseilleur à la cour de Savoie." See Pineaux, *La Poésie des Protestants de langue française, du premier synode national jusqu'à la proclamation de l'édit de Nantes*, Paris, Librairie C. Klincksieck, 1971, 414.

68. Pouchelle noted the presence of dietary regulation in *La Chirurgie de Maître Henri de Mondeville* (1306), and affirmed that "Les médecins en effet avaient, d'après Mondeville, la continuelle préoccupation de 'veiller à la cuisine,' " 124.

69. The theme of devouring worms was often used to signify the sin of gourmandise. It is prominent in late Medieval works and the works of Clément Marot during the early sixteenth century. See for example Alain de Lille's *De arte praedicatoria*, among others studied by Pouchelle, 284–291.

70. Thomas Sebillet remarked on the *huitain* in his *Art poétique* (1548) that "Le huittain estoit frequent aus anciens, et est aujourd'huy fort usité entre lés jeunes aussy, pource qu'il ha je ne sais quel accomplissement de sentence et de mesure qui touche vivement l'aureille." See *Art poétique françoys*, éd. crit., Felix Gaiffe, Paris, Edouard Cornély, et cie., 1910, 108.

71. The term gender rather than sex is used to mark dissociation from a biologically-based view of sexual difference, and to suggest that the construction of "masculine" and "feminine" roles is a matter of social convention, and therefore to some degree culturally motivated, rather than essentially given.

72. Aristotle treated gender as a class distinction, and as such it is difficult to map

onto the biological body.

73. Some of this may, of course, be attributed to the fact that anatomies of women were much less frequent than anatomies of men during the Renaissance.

74. See note 22.

75. See Lynn Thorndike, *The History of Magic and Experimental Science*, New York and London, Columbia University Press, fourth printing, 1966, Vol. V, 475–76.

76. Paré noted that: ''Aristote, livre 4, chapitre 4, *De generatione animal.*, pense qu'il se fait des jumeaux ou plusieurs enfans d'une ventree de mesme sorte qu'un sixieme doigt en la main, à sçavoir pour la redondance de la matiere, laquelle estant en grande abondance, si elle vient à de diviser en deux, il se fait des jumeaux. . . . '' He added: ''des hermafrodites . . . viennent aussi de superabondance de matiere.'' See Ambroise Paré, *Des Monstres et prodiges*, éd., Jean Céard, Genève, Librairie Droz, 1971, 22–23.

77. This phenomenon is studied by Elena Ciletti in ''Patriarchal Ideology in the Renaissance Iconography of Judith.'' She discusses Heinrich Kramer's and Jacob Sprenger's conclusions in *Maleus Maleficarum* that because women were ''feebler in both mind and body, it is not surprising that they should come more under the spell of witchcraft, which itself comes from carnal lust, which in women is insatiable. . . . Wherefore for the sake of fulfilling their lusts they consort with devils.'' *Refiguring Woman Perspectives on Gender and the Italian Renaissance*, eds. Marilyn Miguel and Juliana Schiesari, Ithaca and London, Cornell University Press, 53. On the theory of the relations between demons and witches, see Thorndike, Vol. V, 69–70.

78. This expression frequently denoted sexual orgasm.

79. The kidneys were thought to have had a role in purifying sperm. See Thorndike. Vol. V, 47.

80. The belief that men could be transformed into werwolves was supported by Jean Bodin in his work *Démonomanie* (1580). See Thorndike, Vol. VI, 526. Paré lists ''werwolf'' (*loup-garou*) among maladies deriving from names of animals. The affliction was called ''Loup-garou, parce que les malades vont de nuict, et hurlent comme des chiens et loups.'' *Oeuvres*, ''Introduction à la Chirurgie'' Ch. 21, 82. Another interesting aspect of wolves found in Paré's works is the idea that wolves taught combat tactics to men, ''Les loups ont monstré à faire la guerre aux hommes: ils se mettent en troupes, et demeurent en embuscades à l'entrée d'un village. Il y en a un qui entre dedans pour donner l'alarme aux chiens, puis recourt vers ses freres et compagnons, et les chiens aprés: et lors qu'ils les a passés, retourne vers les chiens, leur faisant teste: cependant l'embuscade descoche, et prennent chacun un chien, et luy couppent la gorge, et le mangent.'' In Paré, *Oeuvres*, ''Le Livre des animaux, et de l'excellence de l'homme,'' Ch. 16, 752.

81. Bellenger remarks on Du Bartas' presentation of the idea found in Pythagoras that sperm ''étoit un écoulement de la matière du cerveau; c'éstoit un assemblage

de molécules nerveuses selon Alcméon, ou une portion de la moelle épinière selon Platon.'' See *La Semaine*, 281. There was considerable debate during the Renaissance over the theories of Aristotle and Galen regarding the place where sperm is generated. See Thorndike, Vol. V, 46–47, and Paré, ''De la génération,'' Ch. X, 651.

82. The quotations from *Les Regrets* in this section are from Joachim Du Bellay, *Les Regrets et autres oeuvres poétiques*, texte établie par J. Jolliffe, introduit et commenté par M.A. Screech, Geneva, Librairie Droz, 1966. I have also consulted Joachim Du Bellay, *The Regrets*, trans. C.H. Sisson, Manchester, Carcanet Press, 1984.

83. Hippocrates postulated the concept that the body was composed of four humors derived from the four primary elements (fire, water, air, earth). A proper balance of the four was necessary for health.

> The body of man has in itself blood, phlegm, yellow bile, and black bile; these make up the nature of the body, and through these he feels pain or enjoys health. Now he enjoys the most perfect health when these elements are duly proportioned to one another in respect of compounding power and bulk, and when they are perfectly mingled. Pain is felt when one of these elements is in defect or excess, or is isolated in the body without being compounded in the body with all the others.

Quoted by Bridget Gellert Lyons, *Voices of Melancholy. Studies in literary treatments of melancholy in Renaissance England*, London, Routledge & Kegan Paul, 1971, 1–2.

The humoral theory may be further defined as follows: ''The body has four fluids, or ''humors'' (compare the Latin *humere*, to flow or be wet), a preponderance of any one of which affects the physique and the mind in certain recognized ways; and each of these humors is associated with a certain planet, constellation of the zodiac, hours, days, seasons, colors, metals, diseases, time of life and special situations and events, professions, vocations, and the like.'' John W. Draper, *The Humors & Shakespeare's Characters*, New York, AMS Press Inc., 1975, 11.

84. Gregory David de Rocher comments on the theory of the humors found in Laurent Joubert's *Popular Errors*, (1578), in which ''Blood was related to heat (fire), black bile to cold (air), mucus to moisture (water), and yellow bile to dryness (earth). Combinations of these formed the four basic personality types: yellow bile + black bile = melancholic; black bile + mucus = phlegmatic; mucus + blood = sanguine; and blood + yellow bile = choleric, thus closing the circle of the four elements.'' See *Popular Errors*, Trans. Gregory David de Rocher, Tuscaloosa and London, The University of Alabama Press, 1989, 322.

The complexions, ''whence spring all natural actions,'' are also discussed in *Popular Errors*. Joubert states that ''we say there are but nine complexions: one tempered and without any excesses, and the others, which are excessive in some simple quality (such as heat, cold, moisture, dryness) or double quality (such as heat and dryness, heat and moisture, cold and dryness, cold and moisture),'' 144.

85. Du Bellay's *Regrets* is not an accurate autobiography or self-portraiture, nor do I treat it as such. Instead, I examine the poet's creation of a melancholic poetic *persona* in the sonnet sequence. George Hugo Tucker warns against the

temptation to confuse the "man who is the poet with his poetic image." *The Poet's Odyssey: Joachim Du Bellay and the "Antiquitez de Rome"*, Oxford, Clarendon Press, 1990, 17. Henri Weber also notes that "Du Bellay reste toujours un artiste, qui stylise l'impression pour la plier aux exigences d'une forme savante et complexe: le sonnet." *La Création poétique au XVIe siècle en France de Maurice Scève à Agrippa d'Aubigné*, Paris, Librairie Nizet, 1955, 400.

86. Albertus Magnus gives a description of the melancholy planet Saturn, which is the most distant planet, and by nature cold and dry. It is an "enemy to mankind," and especially powerful on Saturdays. *The Book of Secrets of Albertus Magnus*, edited by M.R. Best and F.H. Brightman, Oxford, 1973, 66.

87. Thomas M. Greene, *The Light in Troy: Imitation and Discovery in Renaissance Poetry*, New Haven and London, Yale University Press, 1982, 220.

88. Jean-Claude Moisan acknowledges that "toute la vision de du Bellay, à l'instar du poète pétrarquiste, est concentrée sur ses propres malheurs." "Théorie et pratique dans les *Regrets* de du Bellay," in *Renaissance et Réforme,* Toronto, Vol. 13, 1977, 50. Petrarch's prose and poetry displays a preoccupation with melancholy. Although he does not use the medically derived term, he uses *accidia* (from the Greek akedia, "non-caring") to denote his morose disposition. See Noel L. Brann, "Melancholy and the divine frenzies in the French Pléiade: their conflicting roles in the art of *beaux exercices spirituels*," in *Journal of Medieval and Renaissance Studies*, Vol. 9, No. 1, Spring, 1979, 81–100.

89. Melancholy originally meant both a disease and a temperament. As a disease, it was also known as the cold and dry disease, since black bile was associated with those two qualities. Stanley W. Jackson remarks on the Hippocratic theory that the disorder was associated with "aversion to food, despondency, sleeplessness, irritability, restlessness." Hippocrates also noted that prolonged fear and sorrow were symptoms of melancholia, and that patients suffering from melancholia were "fearful, sad, misanthropic and tired of life." See "Melancholia and the Waning of the Humoral Theory," in *Journal of the History of Medicine and Allied Sciences*, No. 3, Vol. XXXIII, July, 1978, 367.

90. Although I have not used psychoanalysis as a methodological approach in this study, it is important to note that Sigmund Freud's essay "Mourning and Melancholia" is useful because it further defines and separates the categories of melancholia as a clinical and cultural phenomenon. The definition of melancholia, according to Freud, "fluctuates even in descriptive psychiatry, takes on various clinical forms the grouping together of which into a single unity does not seem to be established with certainty; and some of these forms suggest somatic rather than psychogenic affections." "Mourning and Melancholia," in *The Standard Edition of the Complete Psychological Works*, trans. J. Strachey, London, Hogarth, 1953–1974, XIV, 243.

Juliana Schiesari, in her book *The Gendering of Melancholia: Feminism, Psychoanalysis, and the Symbolics of Loss in Renaissance Literature*, Ithaca and London, Cornell University Press, 1992, succinctly demonstrates the pertinence of Freud's essay to Renaissance discourse on melancholia.

91. See Rudolf and Margot Wittkower, *Born Under Saturn: The Character and Conduct of Artists: A Documented History from Antiquity to the French Revolution*, London, Weidenfeld and Nicolson, 1963, 103. The Wittkowers state that "It was Aristotle who first postulated a connection between the melancholic humour and outstanding talent in the arts and sciences. 'All extraordinary men distinguished in philosophy, politics, poetry, and the arts,' he maintained, 'are evidently melancholic'" 102. For Ficino's commentary on *furor divinus* found in *Commentarium Phaedrum*, see *Marsilio Ficino and the Phaedran Charisteer*, ed. Allen, Berkeley, Los Angeles, London, University of California Press, 1981, 65–129.

92. "Les *Regrets*, de Du Bellay, satire et élégie?", *Neophilologus*, Amsterdam, Vol. LVII, No. 2, April, 1973, 149.

93. The purpose of satire, according to Du Bellay, is found in the lists of recommended genres in the *Deffence*, Book, II, Chapter IV, under the classification "Quelz genres de poëmes doit elire le poëte Francoys," in which he says that satire is used to "taxer modestement les vices de ton tens". *La Deffence et Illustration*, ed. Henri Chamard, Paris, Didier, 1970, 119.

94. The brooding pose of Melancholy and the absorbed Scholar are found in an allegorical figuration from the *Divers Jeux Rustiques*. This constitutes Du Bellay's only lexical use of *mélancholie* in his poetry. "Est la Mélancholie au sourcil enfonsé, / L'Estude tenant l'oeil sur le livre abbaissé" ("Hymne de la Surdité," vv. 233–34), Joachim Du Bellay, *Divers Jeux Rustiques*, ed. V.L. Saulnier, Geneva, Droz, 1965, 187.

95. In his *Du Bellay et le sacré*, Paris, Gallimard, 1978, 11–12, Gadoffre comments on the "mélancholie stylisée," and also on the importance of the theme of melancholy in Renaissance humanism, which "dans la typologie humaniste . . . est partie intégrante du statut de l'intellectuel, et plus particulièrement du poète."

96. Because of space restraints, I have not examined in any detail the final sixty sonnets, which were presumably written after Du Bellay returned to France. Rosamond Bovey calls them "an integral part of a text that satirizes the persona of the poet." "Joachim Du Bellay's *Regrets* and the Satire of the Poet," in *L'Esprit Créateur*, Vol. XIX, No. 3, Fall 1979, 39.

97. C.H. Sisson, 14.

98. *The Cornucopian Text: Problems of Writing in the French Renaissance*, Oxford, The Clarendon Press, 1979, 150.

99. "Car selon les tesmoignages des Medecins, . . . l'humeur melancholique se purge par les yeux: lesquels semblablement deviennent souventefois fort challieux, & fort sales à cause des rheumes & diverses humeurs qui tombent sur eux." Pierre de La Primaudaye, *Suite de l'Académie françoise*, Réimpression de l'édition de Paris, 1580, Genève, Slatkine Reprints, 1972, 50f.

100. Although the quatrains of this sonnet are a translation of a poem by Navagero, the subject matter of the tercets digresses from it and presents material that was common in Renaissance love poetry. See Jolliffe & Screech, 120. The

physiology of tear production was a common theme in lyric poetry, and used by Petrarch and numerous French, Italian and Spanish Renaissance poets. For example, Maurice Scève's *Délie*, dizain 369, associated the theme directly with melancholy, which he probably derived from Ficino's theory of love. See I.D. McFarlane, *The 'Délie' of Maurice Scève*, Cambridge, Cambridge University Press, 1966, 369, 463.

101. Robert Burton, *The Anatomy of Melancholy: What it is, with all the Kinds, Causes, Symptomes, Prognostikes & Severall Cures of it*, ed. Holbrook Jackson, New York, Vintage Books, 1977, 382–83. Although Burton's work was not published until 1621, it is useful since it represents a comprehensive presentation of the medical and philosophical thought regarding melancholy up to the second quarter of the seventeenth century.

102. Pseudo-Aristotle, *Secreta Secretorum*, Early English Text Society, London, 1898, 28.

103. In appearance, the melancholic type was characterized as being thin, owing to the dryness of his body. This dryness, as well as making him look wrinkled, causes his hair to fall out and his nails to grow crooked. Galen, *Hippocrates de Natura Hominis Liber Primus et Galeni in eum commentarius*, in *Claudii Galeni Opera Omnia*, edited by Carolus Gottlob Kuhn, 20 vols., Leipzig, 1821–33, vol. XV, Chapter 38, 43.

104. Michel Deguy studies the lack of positive formulae "avec l'anaphore, quatorze fois, du "je n'écris point" in the construction of this pivotal sonnet, which appears midway through the sequence, in *Tombeau de Du Bellay*, Paris, Gallimard, 1973, 80.

105. Cotgrave defines *langoureux* as "Languishing, drooping, pining, faint, failing in strength, drayned of (naturall) moisture, deprived of vigor."

106. Greene, *Light in Troy*, 221.

107. Burton, *The Anatomy*, i, 20, and 242f.

108. See Burton, i, 20, and the subsequent sections on cures for melancholy. "Let him not be alone or idle (in any kind of melancholy), but still accompanied with such friends and familiars he most affects, neatly dressed, washed, and combed, according to his ability at least, in clean sweet linen, spruce, handsome, decent, and good apparel; for nothing sooner dejects a man than want, squalor, and nastiness, foul or old clothes out of fashion." 236f.

109. In fact, Du Bellay considered idleness to be a vice, "L'oysiveté qui est mere des vices." (*Entreprise du roy-dauphin*, v. 27).

110. Burton stated that "opposite to exercise is idleness (the badge of gentry) or want of exercise, the bane of body and mind . . . " 242.

111. "[to escape the ennui of idleness by a leisurely kind of employment], with Vectius in Macrobius, 'atque otium in utile verterem negotium'[and so turn leisure to good account]." Burton thus acknowledged that writing was a cure for

melancholy. i, 20.

112. Burton describes a number of similar cures for melancholy in *The Anatomy.* Fundamentally they involve curing like with like: "as he that is stung with a scorpion, I would expel *clavum clavo* [a nail with a nail], comfort one sorrow with another, idleness with idleness, *ut ex vipera theriacum* [as an antidote out of a serpent's venom], make an antidote out of that which was the prime cause of my disease," i, 21.

113. Marsilio Ficino also studied the problems of the scholar in *De Vita Libri Tres*, Basel, 1561. See Book I, Chs. V and VI. This work was first produced in 1482–89.

114. These symptoms are noted by Robert Burton in *The Anatomy*, in which he discusses symptoms or signs of melancholy in the body. Burton notes that Montaltus, in *cap.* 21, "puts fixed eyes and much twinkling of their eyes for a sign, and so doth Avicenna, 'occulos habentes palpitantes, trauli, vehementer rubicundi, etc., lib. 3, fen. I, tract. 4, *cap.* 18.' They stut most part, which he took out of Hippocrates' Aphorisms. Rhasis makes 'headache and a binding heaviness' for a principal token" 383.

115. In addition, Galen ascribed "studying without recreation or exercise of the body" as a cause of melancholy. Draper, *The Humors*, 66.

116. The indefinability of the disorder often appears as part of melancholy's symptomatology. See Schiesari, 44.

117. The common iconographical representation of melancholia when it was not classified to be of the heroic type was a figure seen in dramatization of the four complexions. The melancholic, "envious and sad (*invidus et tristus*) is turning away with a gesture of contempt from a loving couple, and this figure [is] entitled 'He shuns love-making' (*Iste fugit meretricem*)." See Raymond Klibansky, Erwin Panofsky and Fritz Saxl, *Saturn and Melancholy. Studies in the History of Natural Philosophy, Religion and Art*, Nendeln/Liechtenstein, Kraus Reprint, 1979, 298 & plate 84, "The four temperaments."

118. Lyons, 44.

119. See M. Viatte, "Du Bellay et les démoniaques," *Revue d'histoire littéraire de la France*, LI, 1951, 456–460.

120. Randle Cotgrave, *A Dictionarie of the French and English Tongues*, Reproduced from the first edition, London, 1611, Columbia, University of South Carolina Press, 1950, defines the term Huguenot thusly; "Huguenots, Calvinists, Reformists; those of the Religion in France; (at first tearmed thus of a Gate in Tours called Hugon, neere unto which they assembled when they stirred first; or of the beginning of their first Protestation, *Huc nos venimus.*)" The *O.E.D.*, defines huguenot as "A word of disputed origin -Hatz. Darm., cites the form *eiguenots* from Uiron. de Genève of 1550, a popular alteration of German *eidgenosz* (Dutch *ecdgenoot*), confederate, under the influence of the personal name Hugues. In French, a nickname said to have been imported from Genève."

121. See Robert M. Kingdon, *Myths about the St. Bartholomew's Day Massacres 1572–1576*, Cambridge, Mass., Harvard University Press, 8.

122. Simon Goulart, *A learned summarie upon the famous poeme of William of Salust, lord of Bartas: wherein are discovered all the excellent secrets in metaphysicall, physicall, morall, and historicall knowledge* (London, 1636), 313.

123. Goulart, 312.

124. Agrippa d'Aubigné, *Les Tragiques*, Ed. Jacques Bailbé, Paris, Garnier- Flammarion, 1968. References to the poem will be made by using the titles D'Aubigné assigned to its seven books, as follows: *Misères*, *Princes*, *La Chambre Dorée*, *Les Feux*, *Les Fers*, *Vengeances*, and *Jugement*. Pierre de Ronsard, *Oeuvres complètes*, Ed. Paul Laumonier, Paris, Didier, 1946. Vol. XI, *Discours des Misères et autres pièces politiques.*

125. Richard L. Regosin, *The Poetry of Inspiration: Agrippa D'Aubigné's ''Les Tragiques''*, Chapel Hill, The University of North Carolina Press, 1970, 52.

126. Imbrie Buffum also stresses the significance of Christian martyrdom in his *Agrippa d'Aubigné's ''Les Tragiques'': A Study of the Baroque Style in Poetry.* New Haven, Yale University Press, 1951.

127. See Catharine Randall Coates, ''Reconstituting the Textual Body in Jean Crespin's 'Histoire des martyrs' (1564),'' in *Renaissance Quarterly*, vol. XLIV, No. 1, Spring 1991, 66.

128. Coate's assertion that the lost body of the martyr in Crespin's text becomes ''a point of departure for the impetus to valorize the word to recuperate a new body'' is similar to my interpretation, and might apply equally well to D'Aubigné's poetic text, 66.

129. This portrait of France as *une mère affligée* has been the subject of numerous scholarly commentaries. See for example Regosin, 34–35., and the excellent *explication de texte* in Frank Lestringant, *Agrippa D'Aubigné ''Les Tragiques''*, Presses Universitaires de France, Paris, 1986, 112–119.

130. This theory is found in various Hippocratic treatises that are among the earliest Greek medical documents. See Nancy Siraisi, *Medieval & Early Renaissance Medicine: An Introduction to Knowledge and Practice.* Chicago, The University of Chicago Press, 1990., 104–106.

131. Definitions of the *hydropique* condition found in Cotgrave's *Dictionarie* describe *hydropsy* as ''the dropsie,'' and the *hydropique* condition as ''sicke of, or subject unto, the dropsie.'' Cotgrave specifies a dyscrasic body (*Discrasié*) as specifically one ''Pulled, haled; also, drie, drained, or wrung drie; of an ill complexion.'' The *O.E.D.* defines dyscrasia as ''A bad or disordered condition of the body (originally supposed to arise from disproportionate mixture of the 'humours'), vol. 1, 822., and ''dropsy'' as ''a morbid condition characterized by the accumulation of watery fluid in the serous cavities or the connective tissue of the body,'' vol. 1, 808.

132. Melancholy was classified in Renaissance medicine as a category of mental complaints. However, D'Aubigné considers it to be a debilitating pathological condition. In this, the poet follows the tenets of Galenic medicine, primarily viewing melancholy as a clinical phenomenon and debilitating illness.

133. Ronsard refers to the cloaks worn by Protestant ministers, ''Avoir un reistre long les espaules couvertes'' (*Remonstrance*, v. 203).

134. In the *Institution pour l'Adolescence du Roy treschrestien Charles neuviesme de ce nom*, 1562, vv. 37–40, Ronsard profiles the education of a King.

Ils deviennent apris en la mathematiques,
En l'art de bien parler, en histoire & musique,
En physiognomie, à mieux scavoir
Juger de leurs sujets seulement à les voir.

135. Cotgrave's entry for *Reubarbe* notes that it ''purges choller.'' *Anticyre*, a pharmaceutical metonym for Hellebore, (Cotgrave, *Ellebore*) derived from the city of Anticyre, was a name given to certain plants used specifically for mental disease.

136. Regosin, 20.

137. See Estienne's *Apologie pour Hérodote: Satire de la Société au XVIe siècle*, ed. P. Ristelhuber, Paris, Liseux, 1879, vols. I, II, first published in 1566. Estienne includes a chapter entitled ''Du Péché de sodomie et du péché contre nature en nostre temps'', in which he remarks: ''Et quand il n'y auroit autre chose que la sodomie telle qu'on la voit pour le jourdhuy, ne pourroit-on pas à bon droict nommer nostre siècle le parangon de meschanceté, voire de meschanceté détestable et exécrable?,'' Vol. I, 174.

138. Sardanapalus was the name given by Greek historians to the last king of Nineveh, legendary for his lavish effeminacy. See *The Compact Edition of the Oxford English Dictionary*, Oxford, Oxford University Press, 1971, vol.II, 2640. It is more plausible that D'Aubigné was influenced by Calvin, who in the ''Epistle Dedicatory to Francis'' of his *Institutes* makes reference to Satan who ''not unlike some Sardanapalus, . . . lay idle and luxuriated in deep repose.'' John Calvin, *Institutes of the Christian Religion*, Trans. F.L. Battles, The H.H. Meeter Center for Calvin Studies, William B. Eerdmans Publishing Company, Grand Rapids, Michigan, 11. Also, in 1546 Calvin sarcastically gave the name Sardanapalus to Francis I. Battles, 242.

139. See Ambroise Paré, *Oeuvres*, ''Introduction à la chirurgie,'' Ch. XI, 60, previously cited, where Paré discusses the biological difference between the sexes as one of heat: ''la femme a tousjours moins de chaleur que l'homme. . . .'' A number of Renaissance treatises share this basic assumption: that women are cold, and passive, men hot and active. See, for example, Gaspare Pallavicino, cited in James M. Saslow's *Ganymede in the Renaissance: Homosexuality in Art and Society*, Yale University Press, New Haven, 1986, 81, ''. . . man's natural qualities make him more perfect than woman, since women are cold in temperament and men are hot. For warmth is far nobler and more perfect than cold, since it is active and productive; . . . . And so I believe that the coldness of women is the

reason why they are cowardly and timid.''

140. On this aspect of D'Aubigné's satire of Henry III, Cotgrave's *Dictionarie* defines *sardanapalisme* as ''filthy, and effeminate sensuality.'' See also Ernst Kantorowicz' excellent study *The King's Two Bodies*, Princeton, Princeton University Press, 1957.

141. Numerous historians have criticized D'Aubigné regarding the accuracy of his poetic representation of Henry III. Philippe Erlanger writes: ''D'Aubigné décrit complaisamment les incroyables débauches auxquelles Henri se serait livré avec ses Mignons. Nous nous figurons mal cet éternel malade que le moindre voyage épuisait sous les traits du satyr stigmatisé par l'illustre polémiste.'' *Henri III*, Paris, Gallimard, 1948, 287. See also Gilbert Robin, *L'Enigme sexuelle d'Henri III*, Paris, Wesmael Charlier, 1964, 38–9.

142. For an informative study of the royal body see Louis Marin, ''The body-of-Power and Incarnation at Port Royal and in Pascal, or: Of the Figurability of the Political Absolute''. in *Fragments for a History of the Human Body,* Eds. Michael Feher, with Ramona Naddaff and Nadia Tazi, New York, 1989, Part Three, 421–447.

143. The picture of the hermaphrodite that emerges in D'Aubigné's text and in other Renaissance works reinforces an association of the concepts of hermaphroditism, effeminacy, and homosexuality. See, for example, Saslow's *Ganymede*, 79. Saslow suggests that ''the distinction between hermaphrodite and homosexual seems not to have been rigidly drawn'' during the Renaissance. Ambroise Paré used the terms hermaphrodite and androgyne (man-woman) interchangeably, as did Greek and Latin writers, as beings born with ''double membre genital, l'un masculin, l'autre feminin,'' stressing that ''Les Medecins et les Chirurgiens doivent discerner des hermafrodites,'' *Des Monstres et Prodiges*, édition critique et commentée par Jean Céard, Genève, Droz, 1971, 24–25. The text first appeared in 1573.

On the question of *lubricité*, defined in Cotgrave as *lecherie* it is important to note that Paré categorized men with undescended testicles as ''most excessive prone to lechery''; while those with testicles outside their body were markedly lustful. See Ambroise Paré, *The Works*, tr. T. Johnson (London, 1634) 128.

144. Henry II and Catherine de Medici had ten children. The second son, Louis, Duc d'Orléans died in infancy. The ''second'' son to whom D'Aubigné refers is Charles IX, who was born on October 24, 1550. The third is Henry III, born on September 20, 1551. See the study by Jean Héritier, *Catherine de Medici*, tr. by Charlotte Haldane, Saint Martin's Press, New York, 1959.

145. Works such as these, which were used as formative texts through the sixteenth century, were frequently cited by physicians such as Paré. The principal source for my discussion of the *De Spermate* and the hermaphroditic birth is Peter Stallybrass' essay, ''Boundary and Transgression: Body, Text, Language,'' *Stanford French Review* XIV, 1–2 (1990) 9–23.

146. *De Spermate*, as quoted by Stallybrass in ''Boundary and Transgression'' 18.

147. Note in the introduction to this chapter where I refer to Goulart speaking of Du Bartas' *Première semaine* as a poem in which the poet "proposeth or setteth down the foundations of a Christian physiologie, teaching the Readers to consider the Creatures of God with an eye purified by faith." Goulart, *A learned summarie*, 312.

148. Poet Charles de Sainte-Marthe wrote in *Oraison funèbre de Marguerite de Navarre,* in *L'Heptaméron*, eds. Le Roux de Lincy and Montaiglon, Paris, 1880, vol. I, 76: "Comme elle passeoit toutes celles de son sexe de vivacité d'esprit et avoit en un corps féminine un heroique et virile coeur, ainsi vouloit elle passer le temps aux arts dignes de l'occupation de l'homme et aux honnestes et louables exercices." Cited in Anne R. Larsen, "Reading/Writing and Gender in the Renaissance: The Case of Catherine Des Roches (1542–1587)", *Symposium*, Vol. XLI, No. 4, Winter 1987–88, 294 & fn 15, 305.

149. Louise Labé published *Euvres de Louise Labe lionnoize*, A Lion par Jan de Tournes, MDLV, a volume of her poetic works containing 24 sonnets (one of which was in Italian), three elegies, a dedicatory epistle and a prose dialoque (*Le Débat de Folie et d'Amour*). She has been called "la Sappho lyonnaise" because of her passionate and sensual love poetry, "La Belle Cordière" and "angelic" by one of her admirers (Pontus de Tyard), and characterized as a "plebia meretrix" (common whore) by men such as Calvin. See Peter Sharratt, *Louise Labé Sonnets*, Edinburgh, Edinburgh University Press, 1973, introduction 1–17. The quotations from Labé's works in this chapter are from Louise Labé *Oeuvres Complètes*, éd. Enzo Giudici, Genève, Librairie Droz, 1981.

150. Robert Clements, *Picta Poesis: Literary and Humanistic Theory and Renaissance Emblems*, Rome, Storia e Letteratura, 1960. See chapter 7, "Pen and Sword."

151. Labé, *Oeuvres Complètes*, "Discours V," lines 1189–1195.

152. Labé, *Oeuvres*, "A M.C.D.B.L.," lines 25–26.

153. Labé, *Oeuvres*, "A M.C.D.B.L.," lines 1–3.

154. See "Gender vs. Sex Difference in Louise Labé's Grammar of Love," in *Rewriting the Renaissance: The Discourses of Sexual Difference in Early Modern Europe*, ed. Margaret Ferguson, Maureen Quilligan, and Nancy Vickers, Chicago, University of Chicago Press, 1986, 288.

155. Labé, *Oeuvres*, "A M.C.D.B.L.," lines 26–38.

156. *Escriz de divers poëtes, à la louenge de Louize Labé Lionnoize*, Lyon, Jean de Tournes, 1555, was printed in the original edition after Louise Labé's poems.

157. Gérard Guillot, *Louise Labé*, Vienna, Editions Pierre Seghers, 1962, 114, and 180. Labé, as did other Renaissance writers, considered beauty to be the object of love. Marsilio Ficino, for example, wrote in the *Commentaire sur le Banquet de Platon*, "the measure of love corresponds to the measure of beauty." Cited in Agnes Heller, *Renaissance Man*, trans. Richard E. Allen, London, Routledge & Kegan Paul, 1978, 246.

158. The concluding section of Plato's *Philebus*, 64A-66A, was the prototype for the dominant ways of thinking about beauty in the Renaissance. It mainly consists in the idea that there are three "notes" of Goodness: Reality, Beauty and Proportion, which are "so closely interdependent that they can hardly be distinguished. That the goodness of any mixture must be due to its 'measure and symmetry' is declared to be obvious; and of course the close connexion of goodness with beauty, and of beauty with proportion between the parts of a whole, is . . . familiar." See *Plato's Philebus*, trans. with an intro. and commentary by R. Hackforth, Cambridge, Cambridge University Press, 1972, 132–133. Another distinction of beauty which applies particularly to Labé's poetry, is found in Plato's *Hippias major* (297e–298a), ("Beauty is the pleasant which comes through the senses of sight and hearing.") Cited in David Summers, *The Judgment of Sense: Renaissance Naturalism and the Rise of Aesthetics*, Cambridge, Cambridge University Press, 1987, 54.

159. I have not attempted to suggest that in Labé's poetry the body of the beloved belonged to a "real-life person." Rather, I examine the nature of her presentation of corporeal beauty as a universal value. Lawrence Harvey has noted "there has been so much preoccupation with the beloved as a real-life person that his more universal value as a symbol of the unattainable dream has often been obscured." In *The Aesthetics of the Renaissance Love Sonnet*, Geneva, Droz, 1962, 77.

160. See Wladyslaw Tatarkiewicz, *History of Aesthetics*, Vol. III, *Modern Aesthetics*, ed. D Petsch, The Hague, Paris, Mouton, 1974, 202.

161. Jones notes Labé's awareness of a lack of a "parallel system of desiderata for a beloved" in sonnet 21, in which she lists his bodily attractions. "Rather than describing her beloved according to standard criteria, as male poets following Petrarch's ennumeration of Laura's charms had done, Labé asks instead what the standards of masculine beauty are (what build? what sort of hair? what coloring?)." See "Petrarchism with a difference," in *A New History of French Literature*, ed. Denis Hollier, Cambridge, Massachusetts, London, Harvard University Press, 1989, 214–215.

162. Michel de Certeau, "Des outils pour écrire le corps," *Traverses* 14–15, April 1979, 12.

163. "The Greek term translated by judgment, (Latin *iudicare*) is *krinein*, meaning to distinguish, discriminate, or separate. The Latin cognate of *krinein* is *cernere*, which means to separate, divide, to see distinctly, to select, choose, or decide, hence our 'discern.'" See Summers, *The Judgment of Sense,* 22.

164. ". . . the type of feminine beauty praised by the poets in their catalogues of charms, is, without an exception, a blonde, whose hair is golden or like gold wire, eyes sparkling bright and light blue in color, cheeks lily-white or rose-red, forehead broad and without wrinkles, red lips, white evenly set teeth, long snow-white arms, and white hands with long slender fingers. Her figure is small, well rounded, slender and graceful, with a small willowly waist as a prime standard of excellence. The skin is everywhere of dazzling whiteness, rivalling the finest silk

in softness; and the lower limbs are well formed and as white as milk, with small white and shapely feet.'' In Arthur Marwick, *Beauty in History: Society, politics and personal appearance c. 1500 to the present*, Thames and Hudson, Gloucester, 1988, 68. Notable, of course, is Du Bellay's and Ronsard's initial imitation of Petrarchan praise and their subsequent rejection of it during the period that Louise Labé was writing. See Ronsard's *Continuation des Amours*, and Du Bellay's ''Contre les Pétrarquistes,'' in *Divers Jeux Rustiques*, éd. par V. L. Saulnier, Genève, Librairie Droz, 1965, 70–82. Du Bellay's poem first appeared in 1553 under the title ''A une dame.''

165. Lawrence D. Kritzman, *The Rhetoric of Sexuality and the Literature of the French Renaissance*, Cambridge, Cambridge University Press, 1991, 6.

166. A number of poets in ''Le beau païs'' (Italy) praised Louise Labé. De Magny and Du Bellay were both in Italy during this period. De Magny wrote several poems praising Labé, including one entitled ''Des grâces et perfections de s'amye'', published in his *Odes* (1559). Du Bellay wrote a poem at De Magny's request in response to this poem entitled (''A Olivier de Magni sur les perfections de sa dame'').

167. Ovid, *Amours*, III, 3, 7, ''Ped erat exiguus, pedis est aptissima forma.'' Cited in Giudici, 108, fn. 68.

168. In *Escriz*, 127. This poem is also reproduced in Pontus de Tyard, *Oeuvres poétiques complètes*, éd. John C. Lapp, Paris, Librairie Marcel Didier, 1966, *Troisième Livre des Erreurs Amoureuses*, Sonnet 12, 136.

169. In the *Escriz de divers poëtes, à la louenge de Louize Labé Lionnoize, (Oeuvres de Louise Labé)*, éd. Boy, Paris, 1887, 124, and also found in de Magny's *Les Soupirs*, éd. critique par David Wilkin, Paris Genève, Librairie Droz, 1978, Sonnet 32.

170. Gertrude S. Hanisch, *Love Elegies of the Renaissance: Marot, Louise Labé and Ronsard*, Saratoga, California, Anma Libri, 1979, 69.

171. D'Aubigné, *Oeuvres complètes*, Vol. III, 331.

172. Marcel Thiry, *Le poème et la langue*, Brussels, La Renaissance du Livre, 1967. Cited in William Calin, *In Defense of French Poetry: An essay in Revaluation*, University Park & London, The Pennsylvania University Press, 1987, 184–185.

173. McGowan, 243, ''Finablement, j'estimeroy l'Art pouvoir exprimer la vive energie de la Nature, si vous pouviez rendre cete fabrique renouvelée semblable à l'antique'.'' Du Bellay, *Deffence*, 155.

174. McGowan, 243.

175. Summers, 71.

176. Calin, *In Defense of French Poetry*, 2.

177. Camille Souyris, *L'Aventure poétique: Essai d'introduction générale à une Poétique moderne*, Cannes: La Diaspora Française, 1972, 23. Cited in Calin, 187.

Bibliography

Primary Sources

1. Published Sources

Aubigné, Agrippa d'. *Le Printemps. L'Hécatombè à Diane et les Stances*. Edited by Henri Weber. Paris: Presses Universitaires de France, 1960.

______. *Le Printemps: Stances et Odes*. Edited by F. Desonay. Geneva: Droz, 1952.

______. *Les Tragiques*. Edited by Jacques Bailbé. Paris: Garnier-Flammarion, 1968.

______. *Les Tragiques*. Edited by I. D. McFarlane. London: Athlone Press, 1970.

______. *Oeuvres*. Edited by H. Weber, J. Bailbé, and M. Soulié. Paris: Gallimard, 1969.

______. *Oeuvres complètes*. 6 vols. Edited by E. Réaume and F. de Caussade. Paris: A. Lemerre, 1873–1892.

Du Bellay, Joachim. *Divers Jeux Rustiques*. ed. V.L. Saulnier, Geneva, Droz, 1965.

______. *Les Regrets et autres oeuvres poétiques*. texte établie par J. Jolliffe, introduit et commenté par M.A. Screech, Geneva, Librairie Droz, 1966.

______. *Joachim Du Bellay, The Regrets*. trans. C.H. Sisson, Manchester, Carcanet Press, 1984.

______. *La Deffence et Illustration*. ed. Henri Chamard, Paris, Didier, 1970.

Ecriz de divers poëtes, à la louenge de Louize Labé Lionnoize. Lyon, Jean de Tournes, 1555.

Goulart, Simon. *A learned summarie upon the famous poeme of William of Salust, lord of Bartas: wherein are discovered all the excellent secrets in metaphysicall, physicall, morall, and historicall knowledge . . ./ translated out of. . . .* London, Printed for R.M., 1636.

Labé, Louise. *Oeuvres complètes*. ed. Enzo Giudici, Geneva, Librairie Droz, 1981.

______. *Oeuvres complètes.* ed. François Rigolot, Paris, Flammarion, 1986.

La Perrière, Guillaume de. *Le Théâtre des Bons Engins auquel sont contenuz cent Emblemes moraulx.* 1539, (Gainsville, Florida, Scholar's Facsimiles & Reprints, 1964).

La Primaudaye, Pierre de. *Suite de l'Académie françoise.* Réimpression de l'édition de Paris, 1580, Geneva, Slatkine Reprints, 1972.

Montaigne, Michel de. *Essais.* Texte établi et annoté par Albert Thibaudet, Paris, Bibliothèque de la Pléiade, 1940.

Pseudo-Aristotle. *Secreta Secretorum.* Early English Text Society, London, 1898.

Ronsard, Pierre de. *Oeuvres complètes.* 19 vols. Edited by Paul Laumonier. Paris, Didier, Droz. 1914–1974.

Scève, Maurice. *Oeuvres complètes.* texte établi et annoté par Pascal Quignard, Paris, Mercure de France, 1974.

Sebillet, Thomas. *Art poétique françoys.* éd. crit., Felix Gaiffe, Paris, Edouard Cornély, et cie. 1910.

2. Manuscripts

De Verville, Béroalde. *Les Cognoissances necessaires, poeme contenant plusieurs belles resolutions philosophiques avec Le livre de l'ame, où est faite une description entiere de l'ame & ses facultez.* Paris, T. Jouan. 1584. British Library, 524.b.8.

Du Chesne, Joseph. *L'Anatomie du petit monde, avec quelques sonnets des vices d'icelui.* s.l. 1584. B. Arsenal, 40 B.L., Ye 2623.

______. *The Practice of Chymicall and Hermeticall Physicke.* London, 1605. British Library, 1039.g 4 (1).

Estienne, Charles. *La dissection des parties du corps divisee en trois livres.* Paris, Simon de Colines, 1546.

Secondary Sources

Abraham, Lyndy. *Marvell and Alchemy.* Aldershot, Hants., England, Scolar Press, 1990.

Bamforth, Stephen. ''Béroalde de Verville and the Question of Scientific Poetry,'' in *Renaissance and Modern Studies.* 23, 1979, 104–127.

Barkan, Leonard. *Nature's Work of Art.* New Haven and London, Yale University Press, 1975.

Barstow, Anne Llewellyn. *Witchcraze: A New History of the European Witch Hunts.* San Francisco and London, Pandora, Harper Collins, 1995.

Berriot, Karine. *Louise Labé: la belle rebelle et le françois nouveau.* Paris, Seuil, 1985.

Bovey, Rosamond. ''Joachim Du Bellay's *Regrets* and the Satire of the Poet,'' in *L'Esprit Créateur*. Vol. XIX, No. 3, Fall 1979, 38–55.

Brabant, Luc Van. *Louize Labé et ses aventures amoureuses avec Clément Marot et le dauphin Henry*. Belgique, Editions de la belle sans sy, 1967–1969, 3 vols.

Brann, Noel L. ''Melancholy and the divine frenzies in the French Pléiade: their conflicting roles in the art of *beaux exercices spirituels*,'' in *Journal of Medieval and Renaissance Studies*. Vol. 9, No. 1, Spring, 1979, 81–100.

Brown, Peter. *The Body and Society: Men, Women and Sexual Renunciation in Early Christianity*. New York, Columbia University Press, 1988.

Burckhardt, Titus. *Alchemy Science of the Cosmos, Science of the Soul*. Trans. William Stoddart, Baltimore, Maryland, Penguin Books, 1972.

Burton, Robert. *The Anatomy of Melancholy: What it is, with all the Kinds, Causes, Symptomes, Prognostikes & Several Cures of it*. ed. Holbrook Jackson, New York, Vintage Books, 1977.

Calin, William. *In Defense of French Poetry: An Essay in Revaluation*. University Park & London, The Pennsylvania State University Press, 1987.

Calvin, John. *Institutes of the Christian Religion*. trans. Ford Lewis Battles, Grand Rapids, Michigan, William B. Eerdmans Publishing Company, in collaboration with The H. H. Meeter Center for Calvin Studies, 1986.

Camporesi, Piero. *Bread of Dreams*. Trans. David Gentilcore, Chicago, University of Chicago Press, 1989.

Cassirer, Ernst. *The Individual and the Cosmos in Renaissance Philosophy*. trans. Mario Domandi, New York and Evanston, Harper & Row, 1964.

Castiglione, Baldassare. *The Book of the Courtier*. Trans. Sir Thomas Hoby, London, J.M. Dent & Sons Ltd. 1975.

Cave, Terence C. *The Cornucopian Text: Problems of Writing in the French Renaissance*. Oxford, Clarendon, 1979.

Certeau, Michel de. ''Des outils pour écrire le corps,'' *Traverses*. 14–15, April 1979, 3–14.

Clements, Robert. *Picta Poesis: Literary and Humanistic Theory and Renaissance Emblems*. Rome, Storia e Letteratura, 1960.

Collins, Richard Wayne. *A Toy of Double Shape: The Hermaphrodite as Art and Literature in Nineteenth Century Britain*. Unpublished Dissertation, Ph. D. University of California, Irvine, 1984.

Conger, George Perrigo. *Theories of Macrocosms and Microcosms in the History of Philosophy*. New York, Russell & Russell, reissued 1967.

Cotgrave, Randle. *A Dictionarie of the French and English Tongues*. First Edition. London, 1611. Reprinted Columbia, University of South Carolina Press, 1950.

Dauphiné, James. *Guillaume de Saluste Du Bartas poète scientifique*. Paris, Société D'Edition "Les Belles Lettres," 1983.

Davis, Natalie Zemon. *Society and Culture in Early Modern France*. Stanford, Stanford University Press, 1975.

Deguy, Michel. *Tombeau de Du Bellay*. Paris, Gallimard, 1973.

Diehl, Huston. "Into the maze of the self: the Protestant transformations of the image of the labyrinth," in *The Journal of Medieval and Renaissance Studies*. Vol, 16, No. 2. Fall, 1986, 281–301.

Draper, John W. *The Humors & Shakespeare's Characters*. New York, AMS Press Inc. 1975.

Dubois, Claude-Gilbert. *L'Imaginaire de la Renaissance*. Paris, Presses Universitaires de France, 1985.

Erlanger, Philippe. *Henri III*. Paris, Gallimard, 1948.

Farmer, Norman K. *Poets and the Visual Arts in Renaissance England*. Austin, University of Texas Press, 1984.

Feher, Michael, et. al. eds., *Fragments for a History of the Human Body*. 3 Parts. New York, Zone, 1989.

Ferrand, Jacques. *A Treatise on Lovesickness*. Translated and Edited and with a Critical Introduction and Notes by Donald A. Beecher and Massimo Ciavolella, Syracuse, Syracuse University Press, 1990.

Ficino, Marsilio. *Commentary on Plato's "Symposium" on Love*. trans. Sears Jayne, Dallas, Texas, Spring Publications, Inc. 1985.

Frame, Donald M. *Montaigne's Discovery of Man*. New York, Columbia University Press, 1955.

Freud, Sigmund. "Mourning and Melancholy," in *The Standard Edition of the Complete Psychological Works*. trans. J. Strachey, London, Hogarth, 1953–1974, Vol. XIV, 243–260.

Frye, Northrop. *The Great Code The Bible and Literature*. San Diego, New York, London, Harcourt Brace Jovanovich, 1983.

Ferguson, Margaret, Maureen Quilligan, and Nancy Vickers. *Rewriting the Renaissance: The Discourses of Sexual Difference in Early Modern Europe*. Chicago, University of Chicago Press, 1986.

Gadoffre, Gilbert. *Du Bellay et le sacré*. Paris, Gallimard, 1978.

Girault, Yvonne. *Louise Labé*. Lausanne, Editions Rencontre, 1966.

Givry, Grillot de. *Witchcraft, Magic and Alchemy*. trans. J. Courtenay Locke, New York, Frederick Publications, 1954.

Greenblatt, Stephen. *Renaissance Self-Fashioning: From More to Shakespeare*. Chicago & London, The University of Chicago Press, 1980.

______. *Marvelous Possessions: The Wonder of the New World.* Chicago & London, The University of Chicago Press, 1991.

Greene, Thomas M. *The Light in Troy: Imitation and Discovery in Renaissance Poetry.* New Haven and London, Yale University Press, 1982.

Guillot, Gérard. *Louise Labé.* Paris, Editions Pierre Seghers, 1962.

Hackforth, R. *Plato's "Philebus".* trans., with an introduction and commentary, Cambridge, Cambridge University Press, 1972.

Hanisch, Gertrude S. *Love Elegies of the Renaissance: Marot, Louise Labé and Ronsard.* Stanford French and Italian Studies, Saratoga, CA. Anma Libri & Co. 1979.

Harvey, Lawrence E. *The Aesthetics of the Renaissance Love Sonnet.* Geneva, Droz, 1962.

Heller, Agnes. *Renaissance Man.* trans. Richard E. Allen, London, Routledge & Kegan Paul, 1978.

Heninger, S. K. Jr. *Touches of Sweet Harmony, Pythagorean Cosmology and Renaissance Poetics.* San Marino, California, The Huntington Library, 1979.

Hollier, Denis. ed. *A New History of French Literature.* Cambridge, Massachusetts, London, Harvard University Press, 1989.

Holmes, Urban Tigner, Jr. *The Works of Guillaume de Salluste Sieur Du Bartas: A Critical Edition with Introduction, Commentary, and Variants.* 3 Vols. Chapel Hill, The University of North Carolina Press, 1935.

Huguet, E. *Dictionnaire de la langue française du seizième siècle.* 7 vols. Paris, 1925–1967.

Jackson, Stanley W. "Melancholia and the Waning of the Humoral Theory," in *Journal of the History of Medicine and Allied Sciences.* No. 3, Vol. 33, July, 1978, 367–76.

Joubert, Laurent. *Popular Errors.* trans. Gregory David de Rocher, Tuscaloosa and London, The University of Alabama Press, 1989.

Joukovsky-Micha, Françoise. *Poésie et mythologie au 16e siècle.* Paris, Nizet, 1969.

Kantorowicz, Ernst H. *The King's Two Bodies.* Princeton, Princeton University Press, 1957.

Kritzman, Lawrence D. *The Rhetoric of Sexuality and the Literature of the French Renaissance.* Cambridge, Cambridge University Press, 1991.

Larsen, Anne R. "Reading/Writing and Gender in the Renaissance: The Case of Catherine Des Roches (1542–1587)," *Symposium.* Vol. XLI, No. 4, Winter 1987–88, 292–307.

Lind, L.R. *The Epitome of Andreas Vesalius.* Cambridge, Mass., The M.I.T. Press, 1949.

Lyons, Bridget Gellert. *Voices of Melancholy. Studies in Literary Treatments of*

Melancholy in Renaissance England. London, Routledge & Kegan Paul, 1971.

MacCannell, Juliet Flower and Laura Zakarin., *Thinking Bodies.* Stanford, Stanford University Press, 1994.

Maclean, Ian. *The Renaissance Notion of Woman.* Cambridge, Cambridge University Press, 1980.

Marcel, Raymond. *Marsile Ficin, Commentaire sur le Banquet de Platon.* Paris, Société d'Edition "Les Belles Lettres," 1956.

Mathieu-Castellani, Gisèle. *Emblèmes de la Mort: le dialoque de l'image et du texte.* Paris, A.-G. Nizet, 1988.

McFarlane, I.D. *The "Délie" of Maurice Scève.* Cambridge, Cambridge University Press, 1966.

McGowan, Margaret M. *Ideal Forms in the Age of the Renaissance.* Berkeley, University of California Press, 1985.

Migiel, Marilyn and Juliana Schiesari. Eds. *Refiguring Woman: Perspectives on Gender and the Italian Renaissance.* Ithaca and London, Cornell University Press, 1991.

Minuit, Gabriel de. *De la Beauté discours divers avec la paule-graphie.* Genève, Slatkine Reprints, 1969.

Moisan, Jean-Claude. "Théorie et pratique dans les *Regrets* de du Bellay," in *Renaissance et Réforme.* Toronto, Vol. 13, 1977, 46–58.

Mourges, Odette de. *Metaphysical, Baroque & Précieux Poetry.* Oxford, Clarendon, 1953.

Nash, Jerry C. *The Love Aesthetics of Maurice Scève: Poetry and Struggle.* Cambridge, Cambridge University Press, 1991.

O'Connor, Dorothy. *Louise Labé, sa vie et son oeuvre.* Paris, Les Presses Françaises, 1926.

Onians, Richard Broxton. *The Origins of European Thought about the Body, the Mind, the Soul, the World, Time and Fate.* Reprint Edition, New York, Arno Press, 1973.

Pagel, Walter. *Paracelsus, An Introduction to Philosophical Medicine in the Era of the Renaissance.* Basel, Karger, 1982.

Paré, Ambroise. *Des Monstres et prodiges.* éd., Jean Céard, Genève, Librairie Droz, 1971.

Pineaux, Jacques. *La Poésie des protestants de langue française.* (1559–1598). Paris, Klincksieck, 1971.

______. *La Polémique protestante contre Ronsard.* 2 vols. Paris: Didier, 1973.

Pouchelle, M.C. *Corps et Chirurgie à l'Apogée du Moyen Age.* Paris, Flammarion, 1983.

Read, Malcolm K. *Visions in Exile: The Body in Spanish Literature and Linguistics: 1500–1800*. Amsterdam/Philadelphia, John Benjamins, 1990.

Regosin, Richard L. *The Poetry of Inspiration: Agrippa d'Aubigné's "Les Tragiques"*. University of North Carolina Studies in the Romance Languages and Literatures, 88. Chapel Hill, University of North Carolina Press, 1970.

Rico, Francisco. *El pequeño mundo del hombre: Varia fortuna de una idea en la cultura española*. Madrid, Alianza Editorial, S.A. 1986.

Robert, Paul. *Dictionnaire Alphabétique & Analogique de la Langue Française*. Paris, 1978.

Robin, Gilbert. *L'Enigme sexuelle d'Henri III*. Paris, Wesmael-Charlier, 1964.

Saulnier, V.-L. "Etude sur Béroalde de Verville," in *Bibliothèque d'Humanisme et Renaissance*. 5, 1944, 209–313.

______. *Maurice Scève*. Geneva, Slatkine Reprints, 1981.

Saunders, Alison. *The Sixteenth-Century Blason Poétique*. University of Durham Publications, Bern; Francfort/Main; Las Vegas, Peter Lang, 1981.

Sawday, Jonathan. *The Body Emblazoned: Dissection and the Human Body in Renaissance Culture*. London and New York, Routledge, 1995.

Scarry, Elaine, ed. *Literature and the Body: Essays on Populations and Persons*. Baltimore and London, The John's Hopkins University Press, 1988.

Schiesari, Juliana. *The Gendering of Melancholia: Feminism, Psychoanalysis, and the Symbolics of Loss in Renaissance Literature*. Ithaca and London, Cornell University Press, 1992.

Schmidt, Albert-Marie. *La Poésie scientifique en France au XVIe siècle*. Paris, 1938.

Sharratt, Peter. *Louise Labé Sonnets*. Edinburgh, Edinburgh University Press, 1973.

Siraisi, Nancy G. *Medieval & Early Renaissance Medicine: An Introduction to Knowledge and Practice*. Chicago, University of Chicago Press, 1990.

Summers, David. *The Judgment of Sense: Renaissance Naturalism and the Rise of Aesthetics*. Cambridge, Cambridge University Press, 1987.

Tatarkiewicz, Wladyslaw. *Modern Aesthetics*. In *History of Aesthetics*. ed. D. Petsch, The Hague, Paris, Mouton, 1974. Vol. III.

Taylor, Frank Sherwood. *The Alchemists, Founders of Modern Chemistry*. Reprint of the ed. published by Henry Schuman, New York, Series: The Life Sciences Library, 1974.

Thibaut de Maisières, Maury. *Les Poèmes du Début de la Genèse à l'Epoque de la Renaissance*. Louvain, Librairie Universitaire, 1931.

Thorndike, Lynn. *The History of Magic and Experimental Science*. New York and London, Columbia University Press, 4th printing, 1966.

Tucker, George Hugo. *The Poet's Odyssey: Joachim Du Bellay and the "Antiquitez de Rome"*. Oxford, Clarendon Press, 1990.

Turner, Bryan S. *The Body and Society*. Oxford, Basil Blackwell, 1984.

Wack, Mary F. *Lovesickness in the Middle Ages: The "Viaticum" and Its Commentaries*. Philadelphia, The University of Pennsylvania Press, 1990.

Wear, A. and R.K. French and I.M. Lonie, eds. *The Medical Renaissance of the Sixteenth Century*. Cambridge, Cambridge University Press, 1985.

Weber, Henri. *La Création poétique au XVIe siècle en France*. Paris, Librairie Nizet, 1955.

Wiener, Philip P. ed, *Dictionary of the History of Ideas*. New York, Charles Scribner's Sons, c. 1973.

Wierenga, L. "Les *Regrets* de Du Bellay, satire et élégie?", *Neophilologus*. Amsterdam, Vol. LVII, No. 2, April, 1973, 144–155.

Wittkower, Rudolf and Margot. *Born Under Saturn: The Character and Conduct of Artists: A Documented History from Antiquity to the French Revolution*. London, Weidenfeld and Nicolson, 1963.

Yates, Francis. *The Art of Memory*. London, Routledge and Kegan Paul, 1966.

______. *The French Academies of the Sixteenth Century*. The Warburg Institute, University of London, 1947.

Index

Studies in the Humanities

Edited by Guy Mermier

The Studies in the Humanities series welcomes manuscripts discussing various aspects of the humanities. The series' emphasis is on medieval and Renaissance literatures with a focus on Western civilizations and cultures. Submissions dealing with linguistics, history, politics, or sociology within the same time frame and geographical bounds are also encouraged. Manuscripts may be submitted in English, French, or Italian. The preferred style manual is the MLA Handbook (1995).

For additional information about this series or for the submission of manuscripts, please contact:

Peter Lang Publishing, Inc.
Acquisitions Department
516 N. Charles St., 2nd Floor
Baltimore, MD 21201

To order other books in this series, please contact our Customer Service Department at:

800-770-LANG (within the U.S.)
(212) 647-7706 (outside the U.S.)
(212) 647-7707 FAX

or browse online by series at:

www.peterlang.com